The Complete Book of Handouts for Health & Fitness Professionals

123 Handouts That Can Be Copied and Distributed to Clients

Barbara A. Brehm, Ed.D.

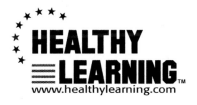

HEALTHY LEARNING™
www.healthylearning.com

The handouts in this book originally appeared as columns in *Fitness Management Magazine.* They have been updated and revised, and are reprinted with permission of Athletic Business Publications.

ISBN: 978-1-60679-100-4
Library of Congress Control Number: 2010922931
Cover design: Brenden Murphy
Book layout: Roger W. Rybkowski
Front cover photo: Jupiterimages
Back cover photo: Jim Gipe Photographer/Pivot Media

Healthy Learning
P.O. Box 1828
Monterey, CA 93942
www.healthylearning.com

License Agreement

Copying handouts from this book indicates that you agree to the terms of this License Agreement for *The Complete Book of Handouts for Health & Fitness Professionals* by Barbara A. Brehm, Ed.D. If you do not agree to the terms of this Agreement, you may return this book in perfect condition to the place you obtained it for a refund of the purchase price.

1. Overview

With the purchase of this book, you have acquired permission to copy and distribute the handout pages of this book, with specific legal requirements and limitations.

2. Grant of Limited License

This Healthy Learning Limited License Agreement ("Agreement") grants you conditional permission to make and distribute copies, as follows:

You are permitted to:
- Make copies of any or all of the handout pages, but any page copied must be copied in its entirety.
- Distribute copies within one physical facility and/or to its members/clients.
- Distribute copies within up to four additional facilities (if under the same ownership) and/or to their members/clients.
- If you are a professional who provides personal training or healthcare services to multiple facilities, you may distribute copies to your own clients/patients regardless of the number of facilities in which you serve them.
- Distribute copies directly to the public and/or prospective members/clients of your facility.
- Print a handout page in full as a page of your newsletter, without modification of format.

You are NOT permitted to:
- Copy pages of the book other than the handout pages.
- Alter the format or content of the handout pages, except to add your and/or your organization's name and identifying information.
- Make copies available for distribution in other facilities (beyond the maximum of five facilities under one ownership).
- Reproduce any portion of the text of the handouts or book in other formats.
- Publish or post copies in part or in full on the Internet.
- Publish copies in part or in full in an outside newspaper, magazine, or in any other medium not part of your facility(ies) or practice.
- Sell copies in any form.
- Make copies available to third parties for further reproduction.

3. Transfer of License

This license is not transferable and applies only to the original purchaser of the book.

4. Termination of Agreement

This license will automatically terminate upon breach of one or more of its terms.

5. Further Information

If you have questions about this Agreement, or wish to request permission for uses not granted by this Agreement, contact Healthy Learning via email at: info@healthylearning.com

For Peter, Ian, and Adam, with love.

Dedication

Acknowledgments

Special thanks go to Jim Peterson at Healthy Learning, for encouraging me to pull this book together. Many thanks also to the folks at Healthy Learning, who turned my manuscript into a book, including Angie Perry, Niccole Deneke, and Megan Comstock.

Thank you to the readers of *Fitness Management* who have used the Client Handout columns through the years, especially to those of you who have emailed or written with feedback and suggestions. I am constantly amazed at the diversity of fitness professionals I have heard from and worked with, and at the devotion and richness of experience you all bring to your work.

Thank you to my colleagues at Smith College, especially James H. Johnson and Donald S. Siegel, who have been supportive of my translation work (translating science into English) as worthwhile scholarship for a health educator. I have learned so much from all of my colleagues at Smith, and appreciate all of your feedback and encouragement. Colleagues from the American College of Sports Medicine, especially members of the New England Chapter have also been an inspiration and source of encouragement through the years.

Contents

Using Handouts Effectively

Handouts may be incorporated into your classes and facilities in many ways. As a fitness instructor, I often bring handouts to class. Some days, I simply set them out on a table by the door. Occasionally, I will give a "one-minute lecture" during the stretching exercises at the end of class, highlighting important points from one of the articles.

Many facilities post copies of the articles on bulletin boards. Some incorporate copies into various types of informational packets for their clients. As a personal trainer, I keep folders of the articles on hand, and find them helpful when answering clients' questions. Many of my clients are time-conscious; they do not want to spend too much of their personal-training sessions chatting (I must avoid my urge to lecture), and they appreciate the written information they can read and digest at their leisure.

Fitness professionals find themselves fielding questions on topics ranging from sports medicine to balancing work and family. Fitness instructors and personal trainers can't possibly be experts on every question that clients ask, and we must be careful to respect the boundaries of our expertise, always referring clients to appropriate sources as necessary. Aches and pains? Be a good listener, but then refer them to their health-care providers. Do you suspect eating disorders or depression? Suggest they seek the help of a counselor.

Handouts alone rarely lead to behavior change. These handouts are most effective when you use them in conjunction with your encouragement, leadership, cheerleading, and coaching to motivate clients who are ready to make lifestyle improvements. Use handouts to show that you care about your clients' questions, and to show that you are willing to go that extra mile to find them helpful scientific information that is relevant and useful.

Introduction

Advice for Beginning Exercisers

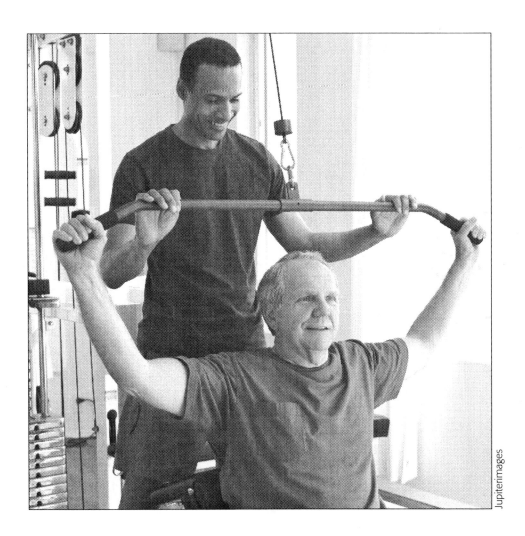

Jupiterimages

Chapter 1

Feeling at Home in the Fitness Center

It's easy to see why many people feel self-conscious in new exercise settings. Everyone else seems to know what they are doing, while you may not even know how to get back to the locker room. Posters of super fit models and athletes might remind you of what you do not look like. Perhaps your exercise apparel feels revealing and uncomfortable. If you join a class that has many returning members, you wonder how everyone can follow the instructor's directions when you thought she was speaking a foreign language.

Never fear! Almost everyone feels this way when they are in an unfamiliar setting. But before long you will feel right at home. In the meantime, there are many ways to reduce your feelings of self-consciousness so that your exercise experience will be more enjoyable and rewarding.

Get the information you need.

Don't be shy about asking questions. If you have just joined a new fitness center, you will probably have an orientation session. Make the most of this time. Don't be afraid to interrupt your tour guide and ask for the information you need. No question is too silly. Find out how to use the lockers, get towels, and so forth.

If you will be using the exercise machines, be sure to sign up for at least one good orientation session or personal training session to help you design a safe, effective exercise program. Personal training is a great investment. Your trainer can answer all of your questions, and help you feel at home more quickly. Even just three or four sessions can get you off to a good start.

If you have signed up for a new class, arrive a little early and introduce yourself to the instructor. While he may be busy setting up, he should have a few minutes to answer any questions you have. Be sure to discuss any health concerns that might affect your participation, and get his advice on what exercises to modify or avoid. You will enjoy class more if you feel safe and confident.

Invite a friend to join you.

Like magic, the environment becomes more relaxed and familiar! Exercising with a friend makes you feel less self-conscious. In addition, knowing your friend is waiting for you motivates you to show up for your workout. Invite a friend who shares your physical activity preferences, and has a fairly compatible fitness level so neither of you is embarrassed about slowing the other down. Maybe a whole group of friends would like to do something together.

Create a diversion.

A good diversion gets your mind off yourself. If you are working out on machines, can you watch television or a movie? Many people take along their favorite music. Music is a great mood enhancer – find tunes that give you lots of positive energy. Some machines are equipped with reading stands. You might find some light reading a good diversion.

Dress for success.

Find workout clothes you feel good in. While some teachers suggest certain types of clothing, there is usually room for personal interpretation of these guidelines. If you are not comfortable in skin-tight outfits, wear something else.

Find activities you enjoy.

You are more likely to stick to your exercise program if your activities are fun, or at least not a miserable experience. Don't be afraid to try new activities, but if you find you dread going to your exercise class or workout, you may be tempted to quit. Decide what's not working for you, and try something else.

Join activities appropriate for your level of fitness and experience.

If you are already self-conscious about working out, joining an advanced group could make you feel worse! If in doubt, start with a beginning level class to boost your confidence.

Banish negative self-talk.

Do you ever find yourself in conversation with your inner critic? Does your critic tell you you're too fat, too thin, too old, or too clumsy? Maybe your body's not perfect, but dwelling on your imperfections makes exercise an unpleasant experience. Instead, talk back. Remind yourself of your positive attributes, projects you are excited about, or vacations you are planning. Be grateful for your health and all your body *can* do. Remember: exercise should provide a diversion from anxiety – not one more source of stress!

Getting Started: First Steps to Lifelong Fitness

Beginning an exercise habit has many rewards. Our bodies were made to move, and movement keeps us healthy. Every part of the body grows stronger with regular activity, from muscles, joints and bones, to the heart and blood vessels. Regular physical activity fights anxiety and depression, and helps you sleep better. Once you make regular physical activity a priority, you'll wonder how you ever lived without it.

The key to exercise success is to start slowly and increase gradually, and to think: "lifelong." You are developing an exercise habit that will be with you for years to come. Try to find activities that are enjoyable and convenient for you. Following are a few more ideas for sticking with your decision to exercise.

Talk to your doctor.

Even people who have chronic health problems can exercise safely, but there may be some important guidelines to follow. Because exercise improves health in many ways, certain medication dosages may need to be adjusted as you get into shape. For example, medication for high blood pressure, type 2 diabetes or depression may need to be reduced.

Put safety first.

If you are walking or bicycling, be sure your route keeps you away from dangerous traffic as much as possible. Wear bright colors to increase your visibility to motorists.

Use whatever safety equipment is recommended for your activity, such as a good helmet for bicycling. Invest in good-quality, well-fitting footwear to prevent injury.

If you are beginning an unfamiliar activity, ask an exercise instructor for safety information. And be sure you are performing the activity correctly.

Start slowly, and build gradually.

If you have not exercised for a long time, you may begin with as little as five minutes of low-intensity exercise per session. You might try walking, exercising in water or using an exercise cycle. Pace yourself, and work at a level that allows for conversation without breathlessness. As the activity starts to feel easier, add another minute, until you are eventually exercising for at least 30 minutes a day.

Add strength training.

When muscles are not challenged, muscle mass is gradually lost at the rate of several pounds per decade, beginning during a person's 30s. Loss of muscle tissue results in weakness, inflexibility and a decline in metabolic rate. Everyone needs a little strength training to keep muscles, joints and bones healthy. Even 15 or 20 minutes twice a week can help you increase muscle strength and flexibility. Exercise with weights or weight machines at home or at a fitness center.

Work with a certified fitness instructor if you are new to strength training. Once you understand how to work safely and effectively, you will wonder why you thought strength training was only for athletes. And feeling firmer and stronger can really lift your spirits.

Keep a record of your workouts.

Post a calendar in a convenient spot, and record your workouts. Let this calendar be a reminder of your commitment to good health. Filling in your daily workout becomes its own reward.

Find an exercise buddy or group.

Many people say that when they don't feel like exercising, if a friend is counting on them, they are more likely to get out of the house. The friend can also be a dog who needs a walk!

Some people like group activities. Contra dancing, folk dancing, and ballroom dancing don't even feel like exercise! Exercise classes with good instructors and lively music can be invigorating, if the pace suits your fitness level. Check out local hiking and bicycling groups.

Make your health a priority.

If you are not used to taking care of yourself, making health a priority may take some practice. If you have thought of exercise as a waste of time, give yourself a good talking-to. Think of your exercise sessions as appointments, and put them on your calendar.

Unless your health is a priority, other tasks (or even pure laziness and inertia) will take up your time. Regular physical activity takes time and energy, but the rewards are worth your effort.

Understanding Heart Rate

Many people take resting and exercise heart rates, either with a heart rate monitor or by feeling their pulse. Your resting heart rate provides information about stress and overtraining levels, while your exercise heart rate provides a good estimate of exercise intensity. Both of these variables may change over time if you continue to exercise, and provide good markers of physical conditioning.

Resting Heart Rate

Take your resting heart rate at your most relaxed. For most people this will be lying in bed, either before falling asleep at night, or first thing in the morning. But not after a loud alarm clock! Find your pulse, and count for thirty seconds, then multiply by two to get your beats per minute (bpm).

Your resting heart rate will vary somewhat from day to day. This is normal, and over time you will get a sense of what a normal range is for you. In general, resting heart rates tend to range from 60 to 80 bpm. Some people have resting heart rates higher than this, while athletes may have resting heart rates as low as 40 bpm or less.

Many factors affect your resting heart rate. Anything that stimulates the fight-or-flight stress response will speed up your heart rate, including emotions such as anxiety, stress, and excitement. Drugs such as nicotine, caffeine, pseudoephedrine, and ephedra do the same thing. Fever, illness, overtraining, and large meals also elevate resting heart rate.

If you have not been exercising regularly, you may see a slight decrease (5 to 10 bpm) in your resting heart rate after a few months of training. This is a healthy sign that means your nervous system is, well, less nervous and more balanced. You may find you are also feeling a little less irritable and anxious.

Exercise Heart Rate

The harder you are exercising, the more blood you must circulate to deliver nutrients and oxygen, and to remove heat and waste products. This is why your heart rate increases in proportion to exercise intensity. Taking heart rate during exercise tells you how hard you are working.

Your health providers or exercise instructors may have recommended certain target heart rates for your exercise program. They want to be sure you are working hard enough to get all the wonderful health benefits possible from your exercise program. If you have health problems, you may have been told to keep your heart rate below a certain level to be sure you are exercising safely.

Target heart rate zones may be calculated in many ways. Your recommended target heart rate zones may have been calculated from an exercise test that measured your heart rate during exercise. The test may or may not have measured your maximum heart rate. (Maximum heart rate is taken while you exercise at maximal effort.) The test may have linked your heart rate to your perception of exertion, how hard the work felt to you. Target heart rates based on exercise testing tend to be the most helpful.

Target heart rate zones calculated from age-predicted maximum heart rate estimates may not be as accurate for you. Predictions of maximal heart rate have a standard deviation of ten beats per minute. This means that at least a third of all exercisers will have heart rates higher or lower than a twenty beat range around the maximum heart rate predicted for their age. While your age-predicted maximum heart rate might be 170 bpm, only two thirds of exercisers your age will have a true maximum heart rate of 160 to 180 bpm.

As you work with target heart rate zones, you will become accustomed to what certain target ranges feel like. If you have to work like a maniac to get your heart rate high enough to reach your recommended zone, talk to your exercise instructor. Maybe you have a naturally lower heart rate. Similarly, if your heart rate always seems very high even with a fairly light workload, you may have a somewhat higher than average heart rate.

With regular exercise training, you may find that your exercise heart rate for a standard workload (for example, running on the treadmill at 8 mph) decreases. This is a sign that your body is getting better at producing energy. In order to exercise in your target zone, you will need to increase the exercise intensity.

Physical Conditioning: The Training Effect

We take it for granted that when we exercise, our bodies respond by getting "in shape." Some training results are noticeable: better muscle tone, less body fat, less fatigue climbing a flight of stairs, or less irritability. But what we see is really only the tip of the iceberg, so to speak. Numerous less observable changes are taking place that contribute to improved athletic performance and good health. The following are a few of the changes taking place as you train.

Energy-production systems gear up.

Physical activity requires energy. Your body makes energy by harnessing the chemical bond energy stored in carbohydrate, protein, and fat. The systems for converting chemical bond energy into energy your body can use for movement are quite complex. With exercise training, these systems increase their productive capacity.

The way these systems improve depends upon how you are training. If you are training with movements that require explosive power (power lifting or plyometrics, for example), your immediate energy system will improve. If you are training with high intensity intervals you will improve both your short-term energy system (also known as glycolysis or the lactic acid system) and your aerobic energy systems. And of course, endurance training improves aerobic energy production.

These energy systems improve in part because of increased concentrations of the enzymes responsible for these biochemical pathways. The aerobic energy system increases the size and number of cellular organelles called mitochondria; this is where energy is produced for aerobic exercise. With training, your muscles store more fuel substrates (such as fats and carbohydrate).

The result? You have more energy available for muscle contraction. Daily activities also feel easier because your body can produce energy more quickly.

With training, the cells become more responsive to the hormone insulin, which signals the cells to take up glucose from the blood. Improved insulin sensitivity reduces your risk of developing type 2 diabetes, a blood sugar regulation disorder. With training, your body becomes better at using fat for fuel, which improves exercise endurance, sparing muscle glycogen (carbohydrate) so you are less likely to run out of fuel during long exercise durations.

Oxygen delivery and waste removal improves.

Your body needs oxygen to make energy. Even anaerobic energy systems (immediate and short-term energy systems) require oxygen to replenish themselves. Oxygen delivery and utilization systems improve with exercise training, so the mitochondria get more oxygen faster.

The cardiovascular system delivers oxygen to and removes waste products from the cells. With aerobic training, your body increases blood volume, so more oxygen can be carried by the red blood cells. The blood also clots more slowly; this reduces risk of harmful blood clots. The heart becomes a more efficient pump, pumping more blood per beat, and more blood per minute. New blood vessels form to supply more blood to the heart muscle.

Your body improves its ability to increase blood flow to the active muscles. More capillaries (the smallest blood vessels, where oxygen delivery to the cells actually occurs) develop in trained muscles. These changes mean that training improves your ability to deliver oxygen to the muscles, and that your muscles get better at extracting oxygen from the blood stream. Similarly, waste products such as carbon dioxide are removed more quickly.

Muscle fibers adapt to training demands.

Energy production occurs in muscle fibers. Endurance muscle fibers (slow-twitch fibers) become better at producing energy in response to endurance training. Anaerobic and power training increase the capacities of the fast-twitch fibers. Fast twitch fibers become stronger and larger, which is why your muscles get bigger with resistance training.

Bones and joints become stronger.

Bones become denser in proportion to the amount of force placed upon them, the greater the force, the greater the response. Heavy lifting and jumping produce greater changes than swimming, where the bones experience less force. Tendons, ligaments, joint capsules, and other joint structures become stronger with resistance training.

Your stress response chills out.

Your physical response to exercise is regulated by the nervous and endocrine (hormonal) systems. These systems become better at producing movement and the right level of arousal to meet activity needs. A side effect of exercise training is that the body experiences less of a stress arousal in response to mild to moderate non-exercise forms of stress. You may feel more relaxed, less irritable, and not jump so quickly at loud noises. But don't worry: if a true emergency arises you will be able to respond faster and more forcefully than ever!

Stretching 101

Stretching—We know we should do more of it, but there never seems to be enough time. And when we do find time to stretch, we wonder if it's really doing any good.

We've all seen what can happen to flexibility as people age. A decline in flexibility can mean poor posture and consequent muscle aches and pains, along with limited and painful movement. Regular stretching can help preserve flexibility, and keep muscles and joints healthy. Regular stretching can also reduce risk of injury, and counteract chronic muscle tension that arises from too much stress and a sedentary lifestyle.

Visit almost any exercise class or weight room and you will see many styles of stretching. Some people appear to be tense, rigid and hunched up, forcing a stretching position that is uncomfortable, their muscles tightening in protest. As you can imagine, this approach is relatively ineffective. Other people sink into a stretching position with the relaxation of a cat basking in the morning sun. These folks are getting the most from their stretching exercises.

Fitness experts generally recommend about 10 to 20 minutes of stretching at least three times a week. The following are nine suggestions for maximizing the benefits of your stretching program.

1. See your doctor first, if needed.

Check with your doctor, and get guidance from a physical therapist if you have any problems with your joints, such as tendonitis or arthritis. Stretching an injured joint or muscle can make it worse, and delay healing. A physical therapist can prescribe a program of therapeutic exercise tailored to your particular health concerns. Most of these prescriptions include plenty of stretching. Incorporate your physical therapy exercises into your stretching program.

2. Stretch when your muscles are warm.

Warm muscles are more elastic and responsive to stretching exercises, and are less likely to get injured. Many people stretch for 10 to 20 minutes after exercising. If this is not convenient, try stretching after 10 minutes of brisk walking, or after a hot bath or shower. Stretching without a warm-up is better than no stretching at all, but be very gentle.

3. Be safe.

Learn safe stretching exercises for all of the major muscle groups. Ask your exercise instructor or personal trainer for advice if you are new to stretching. Be sure you are in the correct position for each stretch to avoid injury.

4. Stretch, but don't strain.

Get into your stretching position and reach until you feel a mild to moderate amount of stretch. Breathe smoothly and hold each stretch for 20 to 30 seconds, until you feel your muscles relax and the position becomes easier to hold. If this doesn't happen, you may be stretching too far. Ease up a bit, and try again.

5. Relax.

Use your breathing to encourage relaxation, especially in the muscles being stretched. Allow your breathing to become slower and deeper as you stretch. As you exhale, reach a little farther to increase the stretch.

6. Keep a positive mental attitude.

Enjoy your stretching as much as possible. Expect improvements to be slow and avoid comparing yourself to others. Focus on your own relaxation and progress.

7. Listen to your body.

While beginners may experience some tightness and discomfort when stretching, it should be mild. Pain is always a signal to stop and figure out what you are doing wrong. Are you in the correct position? If you are very inflexible, you may need advice on modifying the exercise position. Have you pushed yourself too far? Control your enthusiasm and go more slowly!

8. Don't bounce.

You may see some athletes using ballistic stretching techniques that include bouncing, but these are not recommended for most people. They increase risk of injury and may cause the muscles to tighten rather than lengthen.

9. Add stretching to your daily life.

Do some stretching when you are watching television, chatting with friends or taking a break at work. If your work involves a great deal of sitting, stretch your upper back, shoulders and neck several times throughout the day. Remember to go carefully if you are not warmed up.

Do I Really Need to Warm Up?

Everyone says to warm up for 10 to 15 minutes at the beginning of your workout. But are there times you could safely skip the warm-up and get right to work, especially when you're in a hurry? How important is warming up? What does it accomplish, and how long does it take? Following are some points to consider the next time these questions arise.

Why warm up?

A good warm-up raises your body temperature and gradually increases the demands placed on the cardiovascular system. By building slowly from low to higher intensity, your body has time to adequately prepare for more vigorous activity.

How important is warming up?

Warming up is always a good idea. When your metabolic rate increases slowly, your energy production systems have time to adjust. Oxygen delivery to the exercising muscles occurs more easily at higher muscle temperatures. A warm-up increases blood flow to the working muscles and improves the ability of the muscles to produce energy aerobically. This makes exercise feel easier, so you can enjoy your activities more.

A warm-up is especially important for vigorous activity. It helps to prevent the abnormal heart rhythms that sometimes occur in response to the sudden onset of vigorous exercise. A warm-up allows blood flow to the heart to increase gradually so that by the time a higher heart rate is required, the heart has adequate oxygen and nutrients to do its job.

An athlete wouldn't think of performing without a warm-up, since muscles function better at higher temperatures. They contract and relax more quickly and move more easily. The energy production systems go into high gear, and nerve transmission accelerates, so coordination improves as well. Athletes also value the psychological benefits of a good warm-up as they prepare for their upcoming performance.

What's the best way to warm up?

A good warm-up mimics the activity you will be doing, but at a lower intensity that gradually builds to your workout pace. It may also include other types of exercises to raise your metabolic rate and body temperature. Once you are warm, stretching exercises are designed to prevent injury.

To warm up for a brisk walk, simply begin your walk at a comfortable pace and gradually speed up after 5 or 10 minutes. You may stretch after the warm-up, at the end of your walk or both.

A group exercise leader may present segments of an upcoming routine for about 10 minutes, perform some limbering and stretching exercises, and then pick up the pace. Athletes preparing to play a sport might perform a general warm-up that includes low-intensity aerobic activity and calisthenics, followed by a specific warm-up with movements that mimic their event.

Is warm-up always necessary?

Aren't there times, such as during low-intensity exercise, when a warm-up is unnecessary? Low-intensity exercise does not pose the challenges to the cardiovascular and musculoskeletal systems that vigorous exercise does. However, it still makes sense to start off slowly and build gradually, even if you save your stretching for after the activity.

People with cardiovascular risk factors (which includes most older adults) should be especially careful to begin activity at a low intensity that takes 10 to 15 minutes to build to a more moderate pace.

Many people have old injuries that require extra care, or certain areas that seem more prone to overuse injuries, such as tendonitis. A little extra attention to these special areas before and after physical activity can provide a bit of physical therapy and prevent future problems.

When is the best time to stretch?

The best time to stretch is when muscles and joints are nice and warm. Therefore, the best time to stretch is usually after your workout. Stretching for 10 to 15 minutes several times a week will help maintain or increase flexibility.

Don't Forget to Cool Down

You're having a super workout. It feels great to be getting in shape and, today in class, you are really pushing yourself. But you're planning to leave class early today, in about five minutes, in fact. What should you do?

1. Use the five minutes to take a nice hot shower to prevent muscle soreness?

2. Do some gentle stretching to help cool down your muscles?

3. Do as much of the cool-down routine with the class as you can, or walk briskly around the room to decrease your heart rate?

4. Eat a quick lunch so you'll have plenty of energy throughout the afternoon?

Good for you if you chose the third response. An active cool-down is important, especially after a vigorous workout.

What is a cool-down?

A cool-down is a period of low-intensity activity that follows a moderate or vigorous workout and helps your body return from exercise to a resting state. A cool-down is sort of like a warm-up in reverse. While the warm-up helps your circulatory and metabolic systems gear up for oxygen delivery and energy production, a cool-down helps them return gradually to a resting level.

Why is cool-down so important?

Irregular heartbeats are more common when exercise stops suddenly than when it gradually tapers off. No one knows exactly why this is so, but it probably has something to do with the changes in circulation and metabolism that occur following exercise.

Blood flow is regulated by a number of intricate physiological mechanisms. During exercise, the blood vessels that bring oxygen and nutrients to your working muscles are wide open. If you stop moving, the blood "pools" in these wide-open blood vessels, especially in the legs. Not enough blood returns to the heart, so the heart attempts to beat faster to increase the flow. Dizziness or light-headedness results when not enough blood reaches the head.

A hot shower, sauna, or hot-tub session immediately after exercise compounds this problem. As your body dissipates heat by increasing blood flow to the skin, the volume of blood returning to the heart is further decreased. People have been known to faint in a hot shower after vigorous exercise.

What's the best way to cool down?

Repetitive movement of large muscle groups performed at low intensity provides a pumping action that aids circulation. Any aerobic activity—walking, jogging, cycling, swimming, rowing, aerobic movement routines—performed slowly can serve as a cool-down. Do whatever is convenient and enjoyable.

For example, if you've just played an hour of vigorous tennis, 5 or 10 minutes of walking may help bring your heart rate down. After a hard run, do some slow jogging or brisk walking. A slow routine at the end of a vigorous aerobic session helps you cool down.

Continuous movement should not be stopped until your heart rate is below 120 beats per minute. People with heart problems and/or those on special medications that slow heart rate should cool down to lower heart rate levels. Check with your physician and/or instructor if this advice applies to you.

But what about stretching?

Stretch after your heart rate has come down. This is an ideal time to stretch, because your muscles and joints are nice and warn after exercise. Slow, static stretches will help increase your flexibility, and may help prevent tight muscles.

Be sure to pay special attention to those muscles used most during your activity. A runner, for example, needs to do extra stretches for the muscles in the lower back and back of the legs. Use your stretching time wisely.

Why Weight? Benefits of Weight Training

To the uninitiated, the weight room may look like a mysterious place. And until you have received your guided tour by a friendly fitness instructor, it can even be intimidating. People working out alone or in pairs with focused expressions and not too much conversation move deliberately from one station to the next. What are they doing over there?

Weight training is a form of resistance training, which simply means any kind of exercise in which muscles exert force against resistance. Weight training uses weight machines and free weights to apply resistance. Resistance can also be applied with rubber tubes, another person, or even water. One of the biggest advantages of weight training is that resistance can be applied in a measured, progressive fashion. After your strength increases enough to lift three blocks of weight, you add another block.

The main reason exercise scientists now recommend adding resistance training to your exercise program is that, for most of us, nothing in daily life provides adequate stimulation for building and maintaining muscle strength. The benefits of weight training read like an anti-aging potion. Following are some of the reasons you should be sure resistance training is part of your exercise program.

Weight training can help to prevent age-associated declines in muscle mass and strength.

Some of the decline in strength that occurs as we age is inevitable. Studies have shown that people lose about 30 percent of their muscle mass between the ages of 20 and 70. That's the bad news. However, much of the loss of physical function that occurs is due to inactivity and a consequent decline in physical fitness, rather than aging itself. In "sedentary" muscles, cells shrink and become weaker. The good news is that strength training enables us to maximize the size and strength of the muscle cells we have, no matter how old we are. Even men and women who begin strength training in their 80s and 90s experience significant strength gains, doubling and even tripling their strength after several months of training.

One of the great benefits of weight training is that it can help prolong independence in older adults. When muscle strength declines to a point where we can no longer take out the trash, carry groceries or take the laundry to the basement, we lose the ability to live independently and must increasingly rely on others for help. Weight training can make an important contribution to the quality of life for older men and women.

Weight training can prevent age-associated declines in metabolic rate.

A decline in muscle mass is one of the main reasons metabolic rate decreases as we age. Metabolic rate is partly a function of how much muscle tissue you have. That's why bigger people need to eat more. Muscle tissue is metabolically active even when you are not exercising, so even at rest, the more muscle you have, the more calories you burn. Strength training can help slow the age-associated decline in metabolic rate by preserving muscle mass.

Weight training helps prevent orthopedic problems.

In our sedentary society, many orthopedic problems are the result of weakness and inflexibility, which are often shrugged off and attributed to the aging process. But many of these aches and pains are not something you should have to live with. Neck, back, shoulder, knee and hip pain often respond to physical therapy treatment that includes strengthening and stretching the affected area. Why wait until you get injured to develop optimal strength and flexibility?

Weight training strengthens not only muscles, but other structures as well. These include tendons (which attach muscle to bone), ligaments (which connect bones at joint areas) and joint capsules. Stronger muscles and joints are less prone to injury. Weight training also increases bone strength by helping maximize bone mineral deposition in young adults and minimize its loss later in life.

Weight training helps you look and feel better.

Weight training is the most efficient way to improve muscle definition. Many people who work out only two or three sessions per week will start to see improved muscle tone after only eight or 10 weeks.

Safety Note

People with health concerns or heart disease risk factors should check with their doctors before beginning a new exercise program. A qualified fitness instructor can help you design a safe, effective weight-training program to fit your personal goals.

Welcome to the Weight Room!

Moderate-intensity strength training has tremendous health benefits, and should be a part of everyone's fitness program. Following are a few tips to help you get started on your strength-training program.

Moderate intensity strength training is safe for almost everyone.

But if you have heart problems, other medical conditions, or orthopedic limitations (back or knee problems, for example), be sure to consult your physician before beginning a strength training program. Let your instructor or trainer know about any health concerns as well, since these concerns may affect exercise recommendations.

If you are unfamiliar with the equipment, please attend a training session.

Lifting weights incorrectly can cause injury.

Warm up before you work out.

Preferably with 5 to 10 minutes of activities that involve both arms and legs. Use the rowing or elliptical machine, if available, or walk briskly while moving your arms.

Be sure you are in the correct position for each exercise or station.

Be especially careful not to slouch. Protect your back by maintaining good alignment at all times. If you are using single-station weight equipment, there may be a card that tells you how to adjust the equipment to fit correctly. While these adjustments appear to be time-consuming at first, they are important. Make a note about the correct setting for each station on your workout card so that you can avoid having to figure this out again at your next workout.

Start at a fairly easy level.

It may take your muscles and joints about four to six weeks to get accustomed to this new exercise, especially if you are older or haven't exercised in a while. Give muscles and joints some time to adapt before you push harder with heavier weights or more repetitions of an exercise.

Start each exercise with a weight you can lift comfortably 10 to 15 times.

After your muscles and joints are toughened up, you can start to increase the resistance until the exercise is somewhat demanding. This challenges your muscles and joints to become stronger. But don't challenge them so much that you get injured. In general, if you are performing 12 to 15 repetitions of the exercise with ease, it is time to increase the resistance. After the four- to six-week toughening-up period, your muscles should feel tired after your workout.

Move the weight through the entire range of motion.

Lift and lower slowly and smoothly. If an exercise is performed quickly, the momentum of your movement does much of the work instead of your muscles. You are also more likely to get injured.

Exhale as you lift the weight, and inhale as you lower it.

Keep your breathing even and smooth. Holding your breath can raise your blood pressure.

Stop if you feel any pain during your workout.

Reduce the amount you are lifting, and be sure you are doing the exercise correctly. A mild burning sensation in the working muscles is okay, but joint pain is not. Some muscle soreness for a day or two after your workout is normal. Sore joints mean you have overdone it. Reduce the resistance or number of repetitions you are performing until the joint pain has been gone for at least two weeks.

Perform a balanced workout.

Each muscle group has an opposing group; work both. For example, the quadriceps muscles on the front of your thigh extend the leg (straighten the knee), while the hamstrings flex it (bend the knee). If only one of the groups is strengthened, the imbalance can lead to injury. If you are unfamiliar with the major muscle groups, ask a trainer for some assistance in designing your program to be sure it is balanced.

Work large muscle groups first.

If smaller muscle groups, like those in the arm, are tired from lifting, then you won't be able to perform the exercises for chest or shoulders at an adequate level, since these large muscle groups require heavier resistances.

Cool down after your workout.

Stretching at this time is particularly effective, since muscles are very warm. Stretching after your workout will help increase flexibility, an essential component of muscular fitness.

The Complete Book of Handouts for Health & Fitness Professionals • Barbara A. Brehm • ©Healthy Learning. All rights reserved • www.healthylearning.com

Personal Trainers: Partners in Fitness

So you are ready to get in shape! Your personal trainer will work with you to design an exercise program that will help you reach your health and fitness goals. But you will be the one who does the hard work: exercising regularly! If you are new to working with a personal trainer, here is some advice to help you get the most from your sessions.

On your mark—Check in with your health-care provider.

Your personal trainer may ask you to fill out a medical form. This form is helpful in many ways. Most importantly, you want to be sure it is safe for you to increase the amount of exercise you are doing. Second, it's important for you and your personal trainer to know if there are any limitations on your activity. And third, it also lets your provider know you are exercising, which might affect treatment for certain health conditions. For example, blood sugar regulation or blood pressure might improve, thus requiring an adjustment in medication.

If you have any health concerns or physical limitations, be sure your personal trainer has the training, credentials, and experience to work with you. All certified personal trainers have some training in injury prevention and exercise science. Some have a college degree in exercise science. Many personal trainers take special courses and complete certifications for working with special groups, such as older adults or people recovering from heart disease. Ask your personal trainer about his or her experience in working with clients who have your health problem. You should feel confident that your personal trainer has the expertise to design a safe program for you.

Get set—Work with your personal trainer to plan your program.

Carefully complete any paperwork your personal trainer has given you. He or she will use this information to design your exercise program. You may be asked to list health concerns. Be honest and thorough. You may also be asked to describe your health and fitness goals. Give these some thought as well, since the more specific you can be, the more you will get out of your exercise program.

Your personal trainer will probably spend some time talking about your health concerns, fitness goals, and past experiences with exercise during your first few sessions. What has worked in the past? What have you enjoyed the most? What factors have interfered with your attempts to exercise in the past? This information is helpful for exercise program design. You may also do some fitness testing to get a sense of your strengths and weaknesses, and so that you can compare your scores later on to see if you are making progress.

Be sure to bring up any questions you have about working with your personal trainer during these early sessions. Do you understand policies regarding cancellations? What's the best way to communicate with your trainer in between sessions? What should you wear?

Go—Make your health a priority, and enjoy your exercise program!

You have worked with your personal trainer to design a good plan that is as convenient and enjoyable as possible. Now comes the important part: making your health a priority so that you create the time to stick to your program. Write your exercise sessions on your calendar, and treat those appointments, with your personal trainer or exercising on your own, as you would any other important commitment.

Keep an exercise log, where you record your exercise sessions. Note any questions you have if you exercise on your own. Should I be feeling this here? Is my heart rate too low? Make a note of any aches and pains you experience during or after exercise. Then when you meet with your personal trainer, ask questions. Your questions are important. If you are worried an exercise is hurting you, say something.

Don't be afraid to ask your personal trainer to repeat information he or she has told you before. Ask to have the information written down if it is hard to remember or understand. Before you leave your session with your personal trainer, be sure you understand what you are going to do on your own before your next session.

It's important to realize that sticking to a new exercise program takes quite a bit of time and effort. People who anticipate the challenges of sticking to an exercise program are more successful in the long run, and plan ahead for the inevitable challenges that arise. The benefits are worth it! You will be glad you have made your health a priority as you start to see improvements in mood, energy, stamina, and strength.

11 Walking Programs: Pick Up the Pace for Health and Fitness

Congratulations! You have been walking regularly for several weeks. You know how much better you feel when you include walking in your day. Perhaps you have more energy, or sleep better at night. Maybe the little things don't bother you so much, and you feel more relaxed and focused.

Walking regularly has many other benefits you may not be able to see. You may have lowered your risk of cardiovascular disease, and improved your blood sugar regulation. Your blood pressure and cholesterol levels may be better as well. Research has shown that people who walk regularly are generally healthier than their inactive peers.

Studies have also found that people who walk a little faster or a little longer experience more health and fitness benefits than those who walk less. The health and fitness benefits of walking accrue when walking asks your body to do more than it is accustomed to doing. This training effect is your body's way of adapting to the demands being placed on it. As your fitness improves, exercise demands must increase if you wish to continue to experience a training effect. A higher exercise intensity burns more calories in a shorter time, stimulates the metabolic effects that reduce heart disease risk, and makes a stronger impact on bone density.

It is good idea to take a look at your walking program from time to time. A walk can easily turn into a stroll, and before you know it you may be sauntering rather than striding. Is your walking program working well for you? Is it as enjoyable as possible, yet still delivering the health and fitness benefits you want from an exercise program?

Put safety first.

Be sure to check in with your health-care provider if you have any concerns about your health. If you decide to pick up the pace of your exercise program, do so gradually to avoid injury. If you experience signs of injury (such as shin or joint pain), reduce exercise volume and see your provider if the injury does not improve.

Keep the elements of success.

What about your walking program has worked well for you? Have you found a good routine or walking partner? Do you enjoy wearing a pedometer? Be sure to hold on to these as you take your next steps.

Evaluate exercise intensity.

How is your walking pace? Most walkers like a pace that is brisk enough so that once the walk is over, they feel like they have had some exercise, but are not so exhausted that they can't get through the rest of their day.

The easiest way to monitor your exercise intensity is to just pay attention to how hard the exercise feels, including how hard your muscles are working and how hard you are breathing. Walking at a pace that feels somewhat hard, but not so tiring that you cannot continue, ensures you should be experiencing a training effect.

Simply monitoring your breathing tells you about the exercise intensity. If you have enough breath control to sing, you are probably not working hard enough. If you can barely carry on a conversation, you may be working too hard, at least for a continuous pace. (If you are performing interval exercise, you may have periods of exercise when conversation becomes more difficult.)

Some walkers enjoy using heart rate monitors. As you come to understand your exercise heart rate ranges, a monitor can allow you to adjust your pace and get your heart rate into the range you desire.

Expand your walking program.

You can keep your favorite routes and walking partners, and still add a day or two of more challenging walking each week if you would like to pick up the pace. Add more hills to your route (if these are available in your area). Join a hiking group (or start one) to get one longer walk each week.

Try interval training one or two days a week. Warm up for five minutes at a moderate pace. Then walk as fast as you can or jog for 30 seconds. Recover with an easier pace for two minutes. Repeat for 20 minutes, ending with a moderate pace for recovery.

Weatherproof your walking program.

If you primarily walk outdoors, you may need to adapt to seasonal changes and weather. Appropriate clothing can help. Indoor options are another alternative. Some walkers use a treadmill at home; others find a fitness center with treadmills or an indoor track.

Consider your fitness goals.

And add new exercise as needed. Perhaps some strength work for the upper body, curls for the abdominal muscles, and some stretching.

New Skills: Learning How to Learn

"Whether you think you can or think you can't, you're right." –Henry Ford

Have you ever felt self-conscious attending a new exercise class, or having a group lesson of some kind? Did you look around and evaluate how you were doing compared to others in the group? Perhaps you even concluded that this type of activity must not be for you since others appeared to be much farther along than you.

People often report feeling intimidated when trying a new type of exercise. Physical educators have remarked that many people seem to believe that good skill is something you are born with, rather than something acquired with practice. We see elite athletes in competitions on television. This is sport, right? We forget that even elite athletes started as beginners.

But aren't some people more coordinated than others? While some people may have a little more aptitude for certain skills, such as those required for sport or music, most of their accomplishments evolved from hours and hours of practice. Think back to those high school music and sport stars. Didn't they practice and play a lot?

And you might think "athletic" people would be better at trying new things, but ironically, they are often worse! They may be accustomed to learning things quickly and easily, and remember being good at sports when they were younger. If you were always good at sports, you may get easily frustrated when trying something new because you are not good right away. You may never have had to work very hard to learn a new skill. So now as you try to ski, it is much harder than it looks! It will take a lot of practice before you are zipping down the slopes with the pros.

As people get older, they are even less likely to try new things, and less willing to be beginners. They are fearful, embarrassed, and nervous. They may worry about looking funny or getting injured.

This is unfortunate. Learning new skills is good for your body and your brain. It is rewarding to watch your skill improve with dedicated practice. And hopefully, new skills will allow you to have fun and be active. Perhaps you would like to learn to play tennis or golf, or try yoga or tai chi. Don't let fear of failure keep you sidelined. All it takes is a little focus, patience, and practice. Here's how to get started.

Acknowledge that you are a beginner.

It's okay to be a beginner! Start at the beginning, with a group, class, or instructor for beginners. If possible, find a group that "looks like you," people around your age and ability. If this is not possible, at least start with other beginners. Let your instructor know you are nervous but looking forward to learning the new skills.

Relax and focus.

While it is normal to feel a little nervous, too much worry gets in the way of learning and performance. Clear your mind by focusing on the positive, breathing deeply, and paying attention to your instructor.

Listen to the instructions, and keep your mind on what your instructor is saying. If you find yourself thinking distracting thoughts *(I can't do this)* gently bring your attention back to the here and now.

Watch carefully and mindfully.

Watch the demonstration as the instructor or someone performs the skill. Imagine doing the movement. Take in what the different parts of the body are doing, and how the movement accomplishes its goal.

After you have listened and watched carefully, ask questions if you don't understand what you are trying to accomplish.

Practice, practice, practice.

Now it is your turn. Give the skill a try. Several tries, in fact. You will get better with practice. Tune into what you are doing, and modify your efforts to achieve your goal. Keep your focus on your efforts, and don't try to talk (or even think too much) while you are moving.

Adjust your performance as you practice. Is the ball going too low? Angle your racquet face up a bit. Are the weights clanging down loudly onto the weight stack? Lower the weight more slowly, with more control.

When your instructor gives you feedback, try to follow his or her advice. Hopefully your instructor won't give you too many instructions at once. Try to focus on the feedback, and notice the results. Try not to compare yourself to others.

Keep practicing for weeks, months, and years.

Sometimes you will progress more quickly, while at other times you may feel stuck. How about some more lessons? A good instructor or coach can give you helpful advice and feedback.

13 Fitness Success = Great Expectations + Realistic Goals

You can expect great benefits from your exercise program. Exercise can strengthen bones, joints and muscles; reduce the risk of heart attack and stoke; help control blood pressure and cholesterol; improve blood sugar regulation; reduce feelings of stress and depression; and help you look and feel your best. These benefits are not the result of magic, but of the time and energy you spend, day after day, and year after year, putting your body into motion.

Wouldn't it be nice if you could find a faster way to look great and stay healthy? There must be some product out there, some pill or exercise machine that could turn back the clock on those sagging muscles, or take that extra weight off with minimal time and effort. Advertisements in magazines and on television suggest this must be the case. Promises for quick self-improvement are everywhere. Lose 30 pounds in 30 days: why doesn't your exercise program give you such great results?

Promises, Promises

Products that promise fast, unrealistic results create both short- and long-term problems. The short-term problem is that they usually don't deliver as promised. Read the fine print. The money-back guarantee means the products do not have to be proven effective. Weight-loss products also often require some sort of restrictive eating plan. Fast weight-loss plans are especially problematic. Many products have dangerous side effects, and much of the weight lost is due to water loss, not fat loss. The weight is usually gained back within a matter of weeks or months.

The long-term problem with products' unrealistic promises is that they encourage the kind of thinking that undermines healthful lifestyles. They suggest that behavior change is effortless. They promise "Eat all you want," or "Exercise only five minutes a day." Users blame themselves instead of the products when unrealistic results are not achieved. Products that promise unrealistic results lead people to believe that quick and easy is the way to go, and anything that takes too much time or energy is not worth it.

Long-Term Health Requires Long-Term Commitment

As you probably know by now, regular physical activity takes quite a bit of time and energy. And, unfortunately, you can't bank those exercise hours. Many exercise benefits, such as blood sugar control, last only a few days. So, to be most effective, experts recommend almost daily physical activity—for the rest of your life.

How can you sustain such a long-term commitment? Research suggests setting realistic fitness goals and designing a program that can help you achieve these goals. In addition, you are most likely to stick to your exercise program if you choose activities that are as convenient and enjoyable as possible, so that you receive some immediate payback from your exercise program.

Realistic Fitness Goals

If you are not familiar with exercise benefits and setting fitness goals, talk to your doctor if your goals are health-related, or to a personal trainer for fitness-specific information. A good exercise instructor or personal trainer can work with you to be sure your exercise plans are helping you toward your goals.

As you plan your exercise program, remember to make it as realistic as possible. Start slowly and build gradually to avoid injury and frustration. It is better to do a little exercise for many years, than to do a lot of exercise for a few months.

If weight control is your goal, it is best to focus on the behaviors you want to change: eating a more balanced diet with fewer empty calories, and exercising daily. Record your workouts on a calendar. Measure success by how well you stick to your program, not by how rapidly you lose weight. If you lose weight, it should come off slowly, and it will stay off if you develop life-long healthful eating and exercise habits.

Improved Quality of Life: An Immediate Return

You don't want to wait around until the end of your life to see whether exercise has extended your longevity, so instead, look for some short-term rewards. Look for an improvement in daily energy levels, better sleep quality, or fewer feelings of irritability and stress. Find activities you enjoy. Use exercise as a daily vacation, and a way to spend time with friends.

Sports Injury Prevention

Sport and other forms of physical activity offer many health benefits for athletes of all ages. Health professionals unanimously agree that regular physical activity is essential for good health. But unfortunately, sport participation sometimes leads to injury, and every athlete (indeed, every person) is at some risk of injury. Risk of injury should not be taken lightly, as some injuries are serious enough to cause long-term restrictions in your physical activity level.

Simple bad luck causes many injuries. One moment you are fine, and the next you "land wrong" and tear a ligament. But some factors that increase injury risk are under your control. The following can help you reduce your risk of sport injury.

Use safety equipment and good footwear.

Use whatever safety equipment is recommended for your sport: eye protection for racquet sports, helmets for cycling, and so forth. Be sure the equipment fits you well, and keep it in good condition. Replace equipment as necessary. Good footwear prevents injury as well. Shoes should fit well and accommodate the demands of your sport.

Consider the sport environment.

Remove or consider potential dangers. Slippery or sticky playing surfaces may need accommodation. Altitude and hot environments require acclimation. Weather may present challenges in the form of heat, humidity, cold, or lightening. Take environmental factors into account during training and competition.

Train wisely.

A well-designed training program should both condition you for peak performance and prevent injury. Workload should be tailored to your personal fitness and activity levels as much as possible, although this is often difficult in a team-training situation. Workload should be increased gradually to prevent injury. Work with your coach, if you have one, to adjust workloads if necessary.

Many athletes include core-training exercises as part of their physical conditioning to strengthen the muscles that stabilize the torso and prevent back injury. Many athletes also include plyometric and other jump training routines in their sports conditioning programs to increase power and agility, and improve lower body mechanics. This type of work may help prevent knee and leg injuries.

Listen to warning signs.

Overuse injuries come on gradually, and by heeding early warning signs you may be able to prevent more troublesome injuries from developing. Early signs of overuse injury include pain at night that goes away during activity, as well as daytime pain, joint swelling, muscle fatigue, numbness, and tingling. Seek advice from your athletic trainer, physical therapist, or health-care provider.

Take care of minor injuries, and don't return to play before they are healed. Remember that admitting you are injured is not a sign of weakness but of intelligence. Sports injury is not a personality flaw, but a fact of life for most athletes at various times throughout their sport careers.

Give yourself adequate rest and recovery.

Rest and recovery are essential components of well-designed sports training programs. The body needs rest to respond to a training stimulus and become stronger. Inadequate recovery hurts performance and increases risk of injury.

Maintain good health.

Good health is essential for peak performance. Follow guidelines for good sports nutrition, consuming a well-balanced diet that includes adequate protein, carbohydrate, and fluid. Rest when you are sick so you will recovery more quickly. Avoid substances that interfere with good health, such as alcohol or drugs.

Cope effectively with stress.

Feeling overwhelmed by stress increases injury risk in several ways. Under stress, peripheral vision narrows so you are less in touch with what's going on around you. Stress increases unnecessary muscle tension, especially in the postural muscles of the back, neck, and shoulders, increasing risk of injury to these areas. Stress interferes with good decision-making, and distraction inhibits peak performance and increases injury risk. Excess stress also increases risk of overtraining injuries.

Stress is a fact of life, and some stress motivates athletes to train and prepare for competition. But too much stress hurts you and your performance. Try to address causes of stress, and solve the problems that are bothering you. Set feasible goals, and manage your time so that you get the most important things accomplished. Make time to relax and have fun. And seek professional help if stress levels are interfering with your daily life or sport performance.

Group Dynamics:
Choosing a Class That's Right for You

Group exercise classes can add variety to your exercise program, and give you the opportunity to try new activities. A class setting can also be motivating. People often find they do more exercise as part of a group than they do on their own. The instructor, the other people in the class and the music (if there is music) distract you from thinking about how you would rather not be doing these push-ups. Best of all, exercise classes can be fun when you find an activity and group that you enjoy. Following are some things to think about when you are deciding which class to join.

Put safety first.

Be sure the class you hope to take will not aggravate any health problems you may have. If your physician has recommended that you exercise, be sure you understand any limitations you have on your activity level, and discuss these before class with your instructor. For example, are there certain exercises you should avoid because of a knee or back problem?

Look for a class that is somewhat challenging, but not too difficult for you. If the class works at a very high intensity, or if the movements are too difficult to follow, you are more likely to experience an injury. Also, the class won't be much fun! Find a class that will push you a little, but won't push you over the edge.

Your Health and Fitness Goals

Why are you considering enrolling in an exercise class? What do you want this class to do for you? Are you looking for activities that will strengthen your muscles and joints? Improve your endurance? Lower your blood pressure? If you are new to exercise, you may wish to talk to a personal trainer or exercise instructor to be sure you choose a class that will help you reach your goals.

Convenience and Setting

You want your exercise class to become part of your weekly routine, so you don't even think about whether to go or not; going to class will simply be a habit. This is most likely to happen if the class you join is in a convenient location and fits your schedule.

Do you have a choice of locations? If so, choose the setting that feels the most comfortable for you. Note, however, that it may take some time to get used to a new fitness center, so if this is the case for you, you may not feel "comfortable" the minute you walk through the door. It may take a few visits before you know the procedures and layout of the facility.

Some centers may offer additional services and activities that interest you, such as exercise equipment or a pool. You may wish to ask about opportunities to work with a personal trainer or sign up for a fitness assessment. Some centers offer special classes in weight control, stress reduction and other health-related topics.

Would a friend like to join the class with you?

Joining a class with a friend offers several advantages. Most importantly, it's nice to spend some time with a friend you would like to see more often. Second, when you think of excuses to skip class, knowing your friend is waiting for you can make you grab your workout clothes and get to class. Your friend may have similar ideas, and you can feel good about being a good influence. In addition, if you are a little nervous about starting a new class, you may feel better if you have some company.

Quality Instruction

Most fitness centers are particular about the class instructors they hire. Look for an instructor who is certified, and has training in teaching group exercise classes. Ask friends to recommend good instructors and classes. Perhaps you can even try a class before you sign up for a series. Good instructors have plenty of energy and enthusiasm, and a good knowledge of the activities they are teaching.

How Much Exercise Is Enough?

When you read about the health benefits of physical activity, it almost sounds like an ad for snake oil. "When used according to directions, this product can help you lose weight, age more slowly, reduce stress and tension, and sleep better; it tones muscles, strengthens joints and bones, and prevents artery disease, high blood pressure and diabetes," Sounds too good to be true. Do all exercise programs really deliver all of these benefits?

To maximize the health benefits of your exercise program, you need to include the right amounts of the right kinds of activities in your program, including the following:

1. Aerobic Activity

Aerobic exercise challenges energy-production systems. Our bodies adapt to exercise demands by improving these systems. Benefits include improved fat metabolism and higher levels of HDL cholesterol (the "good" kind associated with reduced risk of artery disease). Greater insulin sensitivity (cells respond better to insulin) results in better blood sugar regulation, which also reduces artery disease risk. Regular aerobic exercise reduces the tendency of blood platelets to clump together, thus decreasing the likelihood of dangerous blood clots. The heart becomes a more efficient pump and beats more slowly at rest. Aerobic exercise requires exercise expenditure; we burn calories that might otherwise be destined for storage as fat.

2. Resistance Training

When we apply force against a resistance, such as elastic bands or a stack of weights, our muscles, bones and joints adapt by becoming stronger. Denser bones are more resistant to osteoporosis, and stronger muscles and bones are less prone to injury. Maintaining adequate strength is especially important as we age. Many older adults become so weak that they can no longer perform the essential tasks required for independent living, such as grocery shopping and meal preparation. While some loss of strength does appear to be an inevitable part of the aging process, much of the decrease in strength observed in many older people is due to a sedentary life style. Some researchers have noted that with regular resistance training, such age-related loss of function could be postponed at least 10 to 20 years for most people.

3. Stretching

Adequate joint flexibility prevents injury and chronic musculoskeletal problems, such as low-back pain. Like strength, flexibility declines as we age. Regular stretching can slow this decline and reduce that stiffness that keeps us from enjoying activity.

Basic Health-Fitness Exercise Recommendations

The following are recommendations for the minimal amount of exercise required for producing the benefits described previously:

- Aerobic activity three to five times per week, 20 to 60 minutes per session
- Resistance training two times per week, 8 to 12 reps per exercise, 8 to 10 exercises including all muscle groups
- Stretching three to five times per week

Aerobic exercise appears to be beneficial even at fairly low intensities. But the lower the intensity, the longer the workout duration needs to be. In other words, 20 minutes per session is enough if you are working out at a high intensity. If you are walking at a moderate pace, 45 minutes to an hour would be a better length.

Of course, you will want to be sure any changes you make in your exercise program are right for you, and that you are performing new exercises safely and effectively. Check with your doctor if you have health risks or concerns.

Every activity counts.

In addition to the basic recommendations given previously, daily activity of every kind contributes to physical fitness and good health. Try taking the stairs instead of the elevator, walking your errands, playing volleyball on the beach, working in the garden or playing with the kids. All burn calories and contribute to a high-energy lifestyle that reduces risk of heart disease.

Start slowly.

If you are new to exercise, build your exercise program gradually. You are in it for the long haul—it's a lifetime of activity that counts. Ask your instructor for help designing a program that is right for you, one that takes into consideration your health concerns and fitness goals. Your objective for the first few months is to stay injury-free and healthy, and set-up a routine that's going to become a lifelong habit.

The bottom line: Anything is better than nothing!

Do these recommendations seem overwhelming? Start small! What about two exercise sessions per week that include some aerobic exercise, 10 to 15 minutes of weight work and five minutes of stretching? Maybe add a walk on the weekend. This routine can contribute significant health benefits over the years.

17 Daily Physical Activity: What Counts as Exercise?

Daily physical activity is essential for good health and the prevention of chronic disease. Exercise is one category of physical activity, and refers to activity performed for the purpose of improving fitness and athletic performance. But physical activity also includes some activities of daily living, such as walking errands, and household and yard-care tasks.

When do these tasks count as exercise? This seemingly simple question is hard to answer, because the answer depends on many factors. The following are some of the things to consider when you are trying to figure out how much physical activity you get out of daily life.

How intense is the activity?

As you can imagine, the number of calories burned during household activities varies greatly, depending upon how vigorously a person works. Vacuuming is a good example of an activity that may or may not count as exercise, depending on the intensity with which it is performed. Do you move quickly or slowly? Do you go after the cobwebs on the ceiling, reaching or climbing a ladder? Do you crouch down to get dust balls under furniture?

The same goes for washing the car or scrubbing the bathtub. These tasks performed slowly still burn more calories than you would expend watching television or sitting quietly. But moderately vigorous intensities will help more with weight control, prevent high blood pressure and confer other health benefits.

For the activity to "count" as exercise, you should feel like you are exerting yourself somewhat, or even somewhat hard. Your breathing should get a little faster, and you should feel warmer, maybe even start sweating. Activities that feel fairly light when performed for a few minutes become "aerobic," and are helpful when performed for a total of at least 30 minutes.

What's your current level of physical fitness?

If you are really out of shape and have been fairly inactive for a long time, then even fairly light housework counts as exercise. Your cardiovascular system will find activities such as washing windows, scrubbing floors, and raking leaves to be challenging.

The bad news is if you are in pretty good shape, you have to work harder before daily activities, like washing your car, count as exercise. Because your fitness level is already fairly high, your cardiovascular system is more efficient, and it doesn't have to work very hard during most household tasks. These tasks will still burn calories, but they won't help you maintain your cardiovascular fitness.

Will your activities lead to injury?

If you are considering performing household activities you haven't previously performed, be sure they are safe for you. Some activities may favor one side of your body, like shoveling snow and raking leaves. These activities can also be strenuous, even though they do not look all that hard. People with back problems should be careful not to lift heavy loads, or work in positions requiring the torso to twist and bend over at the same time. If in doubt, check with your doctor. Start with short periods of light loads.

Can you walk more?

Walking is one of the most beneficial of daily activities. If performed at a brisk pace, it has tremendous health effects. Look for opportunities to walk errands, and extend the walking you already do on a daily basis. Several short walks during the day add up to a significant amount of exercise. No time for a long walk? Try 15 minutes during your lunch hour, 15 minutes during a break, and then another 15 minutes before or after dinner. And take the stairs as often as possible.

Addressing Health and Fitness Goals

Busy people are happy to hear that daily activities can count toward their exercise time. However, some health and fitness goals really require additional activity. For example, if you want to lose weight, lower high blood pressure or control type 2 diabetes, you may need at least one hour of moderate-intensity exercise a day. And most people will find that strength training has a greater, more balanced effect than lifestyle activities for toning muscles, and improving balance and musculoskeletal strength.

More Exercise Advice

Stockbyte

Chapter 2

Optimal Fitness: Are You Ready?

When was the last time you gave your exercise program a "check-up" to be sure that it matches your fitness goals and health concerns? Whether you have been exercising for three months or 60 years, it can be helpful to step back, take a look at what you are doing, and make sure you are putting your time and effort to the best possible use.

Begin your reassessment by taking stock of your current fitness goals and health concerns. Compare these to the benefits offered by your current program. Consider your schedule, too. What are the best ways to incorporate physical activity into your life at this time?

You may find that you are very happy with your current exercise program, and that's great. On the other hand, you may desire a change and want to incorporate additional activity into your program. Even small changes, such as adding some stretching exercises at the end of your workout, can increase the fitness benefits of your exercise program.

Of course, if there have been important changes in your health, check with your doctor to get a recommendation on what's best for you. For fitness advice, your exercise instructor or personal trainer can be helpful.

Variety Improves Fitness

Physical fitness results from adaptation to exercise overload. Overload means asking your body to do a little more than it is accustomed to doing. Your body adapts in ways specific to the overload placed upon it. Adaptations occur in the energy production systems, the structure and function of the cardiovascular system, blood chemistry, muscular, bone and joint strength, and in other systems as well.

For example, if you walk briskly for an hour several days a week, the aerobic systems that produce energy for long-term muscular work will get better at producing energy. If your activity requires short bursts of energy, such as in many strength-training programs, different energy systems will become more responsive. Applying force to the skeletal system tells the bones to become stronger. Weight training increases muscle strength, but only in the working muscles, and even then only in the specific fibers within the muscle that are recruited (asked by the brain to contract).

Variety Prevents Injury

The right amount of overload improves fitness, but too much overload can cause injury. Varying the type of overload reduces injury risk, as long as a new activity is begun slowly and overload is applied gradually.

Overuse injuries are the most common type of injury seen in adult exercisers. Tendonitis and shin splints are common examples. Such injuries can occur for a variety of reasons. You may have an area that is particularly vulnerable to injury, or you may need to change the way you are performing a certain movement. Sometimes injury can be prevented with better equipment or footwear.

Adding a new activity to your exercise program can reduce your risk of overuse injury by strengthening and stretching muscles in new ways so that they are more resistant to injury. Consider adding an activity that is different from what you are currently doing. For example, if you already do some walking, you may want to add weight training or swimming.

Does your exercise program have activities that improve strength and flexibility? If you have ever done physical therapy for an injury, you were probably given stretching and strengthening exercises for the injured area. Activities such as strength training and yoga can provide the strengthening and stretching that help prevent injury in the first place.

Activity Can Be Fun

Physical activity should be fun. As you take stock of your exercise program, consider adding a sports activity you enjoyed in the past, or a new activity that appeals to you. Learning new skills and sharpening old ones provide not only new physical challenges, but new mental stimulation as well. Some people find that engaging in a new activity relieves the boredom that can develop when exercise becomes too much of a routine.

Training Smarter: Tips From the Pros

Who says that you have to qualify for the Olympics to be an athlete? While the hours of daily training that are part of an elite athlete's routine are not a realistic aspiration for most of us, you can still apply some of the same training principles to your exercise program.

Set a training goal.

Athletes derive their motivation from a drive to succeed in upcoming competitions. Knowing that your fitness and skills will be tested in the near future can help make workouts a priority. The trick is to select a training goal that is appropriate for your fitness and skill levels—something a little bit challenging but not too discouraging.

Your goal does not have to be a contest, although many people believe competition is the whole point of playing. It should be something you can look forward to. You might choose a race you just wish to finish, and it need not be a long one. Maybe you would like to participate in a fundraising walk-a-thon or an age-group sporting event. How about building up your bicycling endurance so that you can join a group ride? You could even create your own event, such as an all-day hike with your best friend.

Make a training plan.

Design an exercise program that will help you get ready for your event. Write out a week-by-week program that will get you into top form a few weeks before your event. Try to make your plan something you can realistically fit into your life.

Athletes break up their plans into training periods, with different fitness and skill goals for each period. During certain times of the year, they have a maintenance or rest period, which consists of fairly light training, usually lasting several weeks. Then follows a period of building fitness and skills, which is designed to gradually get the athlete into top form for the most important competitions. The athlete cuts back on training for a week or so before competition, a practice called tapering, which allows for maximal glycogen stores and rested muscles.

As you make your plan, apply systematic overload, meaning exercise a little bit more than you are used to doing, in terms of intensity, duration or frequency. Increase overload gradually. Experts recommend increasing by no more than 10 percent per week. For example, if you now walk 2 miles, next week you could probably increase your distance to 2.2 miles.

If you are in good health and have been exercising regularly for at least six months, you may wish to increase exercise intensity one or two days a week to increase your pace. If you are adding some higher intensity work, vary your training routine by alternating hard and easy days. Be sure to have a rest day each week. You may wish to talk to a personal trainer for some expert advice on tailoring your exercise program to your fitness goals.

Track your progress.

Keep a training log to track your progress. A simple calendar will do, or use a weekly planner if you wish to keep more elaborate records. It's rewarding to see how you've improved.

Beware of injury.

Revise your plan if you experience any signs of injury. Staying healthy is your No. 1 priority! If you show signs of injury, try to figure out and correct the cause. Are you trying to do more than your body is ready for? Cut back. Use good footwear and equipment, and trim down your program until the injury is gone. Drink plenty of water, and get adequate sleep and rest.

Train with a partner.

Convince a friend to train with you for the same event. You can work out together some of the time, and cheer each other on. When you are looking for an excuse to skip your workout, knowing your friend is counting on you will help you to get out the door.

Get some good coaching.

Ask a teacher or coach to critique your skills. Maybe take a few lessons to brush up on your form. Get a good book on playing and training for your sport, or surf the Web for information.

Getting the Most From Your Exercise Program

Are you making the most of your exercise time? If the time you have for exercise is limited, you would probably like to get the maximum possible benefits from the time you are able to carve out for exercise. The following questions will help you evaluate your exercise program, and decide whether you would like to make some changes to maximize your health and fitness benefits.

Is your exercise program helping you reach your health and fitness goals?

What are your goals? Goals can change over time, so it's a good idea to reexamine your goals every few months. You can adjust your exercise program accordingly if these have changed. For example, if you are feeling tight from running every day, as you train for a race, maybe it's time to add some stretching, Pilates, or yoga to your schedule.

If you are not sure what kind of exercise will best help you reach your goals, you may wish to work with a personal trainer. Your local fitness center may be able to recommend a good personal trainer. You don't need to sign up for a lifetime of training. Most personal trainers are willing to work with you for a few sessions to be sure your exercise program matches your goals, and that you are doing all of the exercises safely and correctly.

If your exercise time is limited, be sure that you are addressing the most important goals first. There may not be time for the "perfect" two-hour daily workout at this point in your life. So make the most of the time you do have. For example, if weight loss is your most important goal, be sure most of your activities are good calorie burners.

Don't forget that exercise has great psychological benefits. Would you like to feel less stressed, more focused? Regular moderate-intensity exercise can increase your energy level while reducing feelings of stress.

Is your exercise program as convenient as possible?

Be sure your exercise program is as convenient and enjoyable as possible. A great exercise program is worthless if you don't do the exercise! As you think about changing your program be sure to be realistic, and think about the factors that could interfere with your attendance. What kinds of challenges have kept you from exercising in the past? Is there anything you can do to be sure you stick to your exercise program over the next few months?

Does your exercise program have enough variety?

Most people like to include aerobic exercise, strength training exercise, and stretching in their exercise programs. A well-rounded fitness program that includes all of these helps increase metabolism and psychological well-being, prevent obesity and cardiovascular disease, and slow the decline of strength and flexibility that occurs with aging.

Variety can also help prevent injury. Overuse injury is most likely to occur when you perform the same motions over and over, or increase your exercise volume too quickly.

Would you like to increase the intensity of your exercise program?

If you are fairly fit, and have been exercising for several weeks, you may want to gradually increase the intensity of your exercise program. You can increase the intensity of a strength workout by adding more weight. You can increase the intensity of a cardiovascular workout by increasing the level on an exercise machine.

If you are walking, you can increase intensity by adding some hills to your route, if you have any around. You can add a weighted vest or belt, or carry hand weights. You can also increase your pace and/or distance.

Try alternating hard and easy intensities during a session of aerobic exercise, a practice called interval training. Interval training can increase the number of calories you burn during your exercise time, increase your fitness level, and boost your resting metabolic rate.

Should you talk to your health-care provider before changing your exercise program?

Has your health-care provider recommended that you limit your participation in physical activity? Has your health changed since you last saw him or her? Be sure to let your doctor know about your exercise program, and be sure you are exercising safely.

You should also check in with your provider if you are experiencing any signs of injury. Ask to see a physical therapist who can help you figure out what is causing the injury and recommend treatment options.

21 Exercise Time and Intensity: More Is Often Better

Exercise is powerful medicine. Bodies were made for fairly high levels of physical activity, and require regular exercise to stay healthy and strong. Your body adapts to physical demands in a dose-response fashion: ask your body to do more, you get more health and fitness benefits. Following are some of the reasons that more exercise is often better.

Higher intensity aerobic exercise stimulates more fat loss.

A study at the University of Virginia compared fat loss in three groups of sedentary, obese, middle-aged women. The two exercise groups burned a similar number of calories per exercise session, exercising about four days per week for 16 weeks. (The third group served as a control group, continuing to follow a sedentary lifestyle.) The women walked or jogged around a track, exercising at a prescribed exercise intensity. The low-intensity group walked at a pace that felt fairly light, while the high intensity group alternated days of light and hard training. After 16 weeks, the women in the higher-intensity group had lost significantly more body fat, including more fat in the abdominal region.

Why did high intensity exercise lead to more fat loss? The researchers suggested that while both low and high intensity exercisers burned about the same number of calories during exercise, the high intensity group may have burned more calories following exercise since it generally takes longer to recover from higher exercise intensities. Researchers have also hypothesized that higher intensity exercise may have a greater metabolic impact on the liver, skeletal muscle, and adipose tissue, perhaps ramping up production of fat-burning enzymes.

One of the nicest benefits of high intensity exercise is that you can burn a given number of calories in a much shorter period of time. If you wish to reduce the amount of time you spend exercising, try for shorter periods of higher intensity exercise two or three days a week.

A greater calorie expenditure per week reduces risk of cardiovascular disease.

Research in both men and women has concluded that even a small amount of exercise significantly reduces risk of cardiovascular disease. A recent study of over 27,000 women concluded that those who expended as little as 500 to 600 exercise calories per week had a 25 percent lower risk of cardiovascular disease compared to women who did not exercise at all. Women who burned over 1,500 calories per week had a 40 percent lower risk.

Several studies have indicated the better cardiovascular health observed in regular exercisers is probably due to several things, including lower levels of inflammation in the arteries, and a lower tendency of the blood to form clots that might block circulation. Greater amounts of exercise are also linked to better blood pressure, better blood cholesterol and triglyceride levels, less excess body fat, and better blood sugar regulation.

Strength training delivers essential health and fitness benefits.

Strength training improves the strength and function of muscles, tendons, bones, and joints. Many exercisers use strength training to augment the health benefits of aerobic activity. In a study of people with type 2 diabetes, those who participated in both aerobic and strength training exercise experienced better blood sugar control than people who participated in only aerobic or only strength training. Combining both aerobic and strength training not only resulted in more exercise, but in the conditioning of more muscle fiber types.

Interval training is important for many athletes, even weekend warriors.

If you participate in a sport that requires speed and power, it is important to train your speed and power muscle fibers. Moderate intensity endurance exercise will not improve or even maintain fitness in your fast-twitch muscle fibers, the muscle fibers important for sprinting to first base, jumping to shoot the ball into the hoop, or delivering a powerful tennis serve. Training for your sport improves performance and reduces risk of injury.

What are the best ways to increase exercise volume?

If you wish to increase the intensity or volume of your exercise program, it is important to start slowly and build gradually. Check in with your health-care provider to be sure high intensity or more exercise is a good idea for you, and to be sure you are exercising safely. Many people enhance their exercise programs by replacing endurance exercise with two short sessions of interval training a week. Others decide to add two or three sessions of strength training.

Take some time to reassess your health and fitness goals and evaluate how well your current exercise program is helping you reach these goals. A personal trainer can help you establish realistic goals, and suggest ways to maximize your exercise time. If you are new to interval or strength training, working with a fitness professional can help you gain confidence and avoid injury.

The Inside Scoop on Core Training

If you have been near a fitness center lately, you may have spotted large colorful balls around the edge of the weight room, or people doing a variety of complicated-looking exercises on the mats. Maybe you have tried some of these exercises yourself, or taken a class that included some core muscle strengthening work. Maybe you have wondered what your instructor meant by "core training," and whether these exercises are all they are cracked up to be.

They are. Core strengthening exercises have become popular at many fitness centers because they often help to relieve various aches and pains, especially back pain, due to weak muscles and poor posture. Core strengthening also helps to improve balance and prevent falls in vulnerable older adults. Many athletes perform core-strengthening exercises to increase the torso stability they need for peak sport performance.

For many years people seeking physical fitness focused on calorie burning aerobic activity and strength training that primarily worked the large muscle groups of the limbs and torso. While the core muscles perform some stability work during most aerobic and strength-training exercise, they may not get enough of an overload to prevent the weakening that occurs with aging and sedentary lifestyles. This may explain why core-strengthening classes have come into their own in the past decade, as an antidote to years of neglect for these important muscles.

What is core training?

Various terms are used to describe exercises performed to strengthen the deep abdominal and back muscles that work to move and stabilize the torso. Core training and core conditioning simply mean training the core muscle groups with core strengthening exercises that challenge these muscles to improve their strength and endurance.

Core stabilization refers to the one of the most important functions of these muscles: stabilization of the torso. The core muscles help to hold the torso steady and in good alignment whether you are seated at a desk or playing a vigorous tennis game. Many core strengthening exercises have the deep core muscles hold the torso still as destabilizing forces are applied, such as by moving arms and legs, or balancing on a stability platform or ball.

What are the core muscle groups?

Central to core conditioning are the deep abdominal muscles, and the back muscles that stabilize the spine and support shoulder function. Some instructors include other muscle groups in their core work as well, including muscles of the hips, buttocks, and inner thighs and other back and shoulder muscles.

The innermost abdominal muscle, the transverse abdominis, is especially important for injury prevention and back health. This large muscle wraps around your lower torso like a corset. When this muscle is contracted, it compresses the abdomen. You may feel this muscle contract when you blow your breath out forcefully between pursed lips, or when you cough. Your fitness instructor may tell you to "pull your navel toward your spine" to help you engage this deep muscle layer.

Two sets of abdominal muscles called the internal and external obliques work over the transverse abdominis to help your torso rotate. They also help the transverse abdominis to stabilize your torso. Core back muscles are engaged when you lie on your stomach and lift your legs or shoulders. Your abdominals should contract in this position as well to protect your back. When you sit on a stability ball, these core muscles all work to help you keep your balance.

What's the best way to add core training to your exercise program?

There are many good ways to add core training to your exercise program. Some people like to try a special core training class that teaches them new exercises and offers instruction on working the core muscles properly. Many good videos and books contain advice on core strengthening exercises. Classes such as Pilates, yoga, martial arts, and many forms of dance work extensively on core strength. Core training should be part of an exercise program that also includes aerobic exercise, strength training, and stretching.

Do you need special equipment for core training?

Stability balls and other props offer variety, but many core strengthening exercises can be done without equipment. More important than equipment is technique. It is extremely important to learn proper exercise alignment (position) and breathing to prevent injury. If you are new to core training techniques, an exercise instructor or personal trainer can provide feedback and help you work safely and effectively.

Getting the Most From Mind-Body Exercise

Your instructor tells you to tune in to your breathing, to feel the breath coming in and filling your lungs. Okay, got it. There's the breath. Now she tells you to feel your muscles relax as you exhale. Relax? In this position? You sneak a look at the slender young woman in the front row, who is so flexible she must be from the circus or perhaps even another planet. You hope nobody is watching you. Maybe if you try a little harder you can reach a little farther? No such luck. Only more pain as your muscles tighten.

Mind-body exercise includes the cultivation of an inward, meditative state as part of its practice. Activities that have evolved from eastern traditions, such as yoga, tai chi, and most forms of martial arts, are considered mind-body activities. Pilates draws from several movement disciplines, including yoga, and incorporates a mind-body meditative focus as well. If you are new to this type of exercise, following are a few suggestions to help you get the most from your classes and practice sessions.

Choose a class or method that is right for your previous experience and fitness level.

If you are new to the activity, take a beginning level class, even if you are already very fit. You will benefit from the instruction. If health or fitness concerns limit your movement, a beginning level class is less likely to cause injury (or frustration). Many people stay at beginning level classes for years because these classes best accommodate existing injuries or provide a comfortable pace. When you know how to work, even beginning level classes can be challenging. Upper level Pilates and certain types of yoga can be quite vigorous and cause injury if you work incorrectly or try to do too much too soon.

Work with a qualified instructor.

Books, articles, and DVDs can be very helpful, but work with a real live instructor when you are getting started, and then take classes or training sessions from time to time to be sure you are working correctly. An instructor can evaluate and give you feedback on your posture and body mechanics so that you achieve maximum results and avoid injury.

Be sure to let your instructor know if you have any health concerns.

Your instructor may ask you to talk to your health-care provider before you begin working together, especially if you have any health concerns. Ask your instructor if he has

experience working with students who have your health concerns, and knows how to help you work safely. In general, the more experience and education your instructor has, the better.

Discuss your therapeutic and fitness goals with your instructor.

Many people experience health benefits from mind-body activities. Stretching and strengthening the core muscles, and improving posture sometimes reduce back, shoulder, and neck pain. Mind-body techniques often help people feel less stressed, which can reduce stress-related symptoms such as high blood pressure and muscle tension.

Understand your instructor's hands-on techniques.

Many instructors give physical cues to help students understand the positions and movements they are trying to achieve. For example, the instructor may put her hand in the middle of your back and encourage you to press into that area to achieve a specific curve in your back. If being touched in this way bothers you, just let the instructor know.

Similarly, some classes have people pair up to assist each other in getting into the correct position. You may be asked to push on someone's leg, or press down on someone's lower back. Maybe you will just brace their foot so they don't slide. Then you will be on the receiving end. Such physical cues can be very helpful when supervised by a knowledgeable instructor. But again, if they make you uncomfortable, let the instructor know and he may be able to give you directions on working alone while the other members of the class work with partners.

Practice mindful awareness.

A mindful awareness during practice means focusing on the present moment, including your sensations of breathing, stretching, holding positions, and moving. Mindfulness helps you work correctly and prevents injury. This inward meditative state is a goal in and of itself for many activities.

When you find your mind wandering during practice, simply bring it back to your breathing and to your instructor's directions. And relax. Try not to try, and avoid comparing yourself to others. Simply observe what is happening for you without judgment.

In the Running or Run Down? Don't Let Exercise Impair Immune Function

Exercise *is* good for you. But athletes who train hard sometimes catch more colds and have more sick days than their less active peers. Many athletes tend to come down with an upper respiratory tract infection in the days following a big contest, such as a marathon or an exhausting tournament requiring hours of intense activity. Too much exercise, especially when accompanied by inadequate nutrition and an out-of-balance lifestyle, can lead to an energy deficit that leaves the immune system run down and unable to perform at its best.

It's a question of balance. Research shows that moderate amounts of exercise as part of a balanced lifestyle improve immune function. Regular exercisers are sick fewer days each year, and in the laboratory their immune systems generally perform better than those of their sedentary friends.

Is moderate not part of your vocabulary? To be the best, sometimes you've got to train hard, and some sports require extreme levels of exertion. If this is you, then be sure to take extra measures to stay healthy, so that you don't lose training days or suffer poor performance because of sickness. Successful athletes pay attention to the factors that help keep you healthy and allow you to train hard without reducing the effectiveness of your immune system. Here's what you can do to prevent high volumes of exercise from interfering with immune function.

Manage stress, and strive for balance.

Excess exercise appears to exert its negative effects on the immune system by stimulating the production of stress hormones. Stress hormones are meant to help get you out of a tight situation by activating the fight or flight response. In the interest of surviving imminent danger, nonessential functions, such as the immune system, are put on hold. Who cares if you might get a cold in a few days when danger is near?

Well, you care! The trick is to keep general stress levels as low as possible so exercise does not reach the "excess" level quite so soon. Exercise is most likely to be perceived as stress when you are already stressed in other areas of your life, such as work, school, or relationships.

Reduce training volume if you experience symptoms of overtraining.

Frequent illnesses and injuries are often indicators of overtraining. So are elevated resting heart rate, difficulty sleeping, fatigue, depression, and an unexplained decline in athletic performance. Train for shorter periods, cross train, and take more rest days.

Get plenty of sleep.

The immune systems of rested people are much more effective at responding to pathogens than the immune systems of the sleep deprived. Sleep also allows muscles to heal after tough workouts. Regular rest, sleep, and recovery are important components of every training cycle.

Avoid germs.

Germs are everywhere, so adopt habits that will keep them out of your body. Avoid crowds as much as possible in the weeks preceding an important competition, and stay away from sick people. The hands are the most common source of infection, so wash hands often and well. And remember, touching your nose or eyes gives cold germs an express ride to the home of their dreams: your mucus membranes.

Pay careful attention to your diet.

Athletes restricting calories or avoiding certain food groups are most at risk for nutritional deficiencies that can compromise immune health. All athletes should pay extra attention to the following.

Adequate hydration keeps mucus membranes healthy, providing the best operating environment for patrolling immune cells.

Protein is what immune cells are made of. Athletes training at high levels need more protein than most people, about 1.2 to 1.6 grams of protein per kilogram body weight.

Carbohydrate consumed before and during exercise reduces the release of stress hormones that suppress immune response. Studies suggest keeping glycogen stores up and consuming 30 to 60 grams of a carbohydrate beverage during prolonged exercise help protect immune function.

Many *vitamins and minerals* play important roles in the health of the immune system, especially vitamins A, C, E, B6, B12, and folate, and minerals iron and zinc. Taking megadoses of these nutrients, however, does not appear to improve immunity. Megadoses of some nutrients may even cause health problems! If your diet is not always what it should be, a multivitamin and mineral supplement that supplies up to 100 percent of the RDA for most nutrients is a good idea.

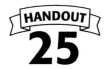

HANDOUT 25 Overtraining: In the Zone or Zoned Out?

The whole point of exercise training is to stress your body so that it will adapt by getting stronger. But there is a fine line between the training levels that lead to optimal performance and those that lead to deterioration (the result of asking your body to do too much). All athletes must learn to discriminate between training practices that give them an edge and those that push them over the edge.

What is overtraining syndrome?

When you place an overload on your body by asking it to do more than it is accustomed to doing, small, usually undetectable injuries occur in your muscles and joints. As your body repairs this damage, it usually overcompensates, making muscles and joints stronger. Similarly, when your muscles have experienced an energy shortage, such as what occurs during intense exercise, the energy production systems respond by getting better at producing energy by undergoing a number of physical changes.

These processes of repair and adaptation take time and occur during rest. When another heavy bout of exercise occurs before your body has had sufficient time to adapt to the previous bout, further damage occurs. Over time, too much stress and too little recovery lead to the development of overtraining syndrome.

Overtraining syndrome is characterized by detectable symptoms. Most athletes and coaches first suspect overtraining when performance begins to decline for no apparent reason. Fatigue, apathy, depression, muscle and joint pain, and loss of appetite are common. Other symptoms include changes in heart rate at rest and during exercise, gastrointestinal disturbances, more frequent illnesses and infections, delayed healing of wounds and difficulty sleeping. Women may experience disturbances in their menstrual cycles.

How can I train hard but avoid overtraining?

To avoid overtraining, vary your exercise program and include adequate time for recovery, especially after hard workouts. Also, follow a healthy lifestyle and listen to your body. Exercise scientists recommend the following steps to prevent overtraining:

Increase gradually.

Start training slowly and increase overload by no more than 5 to 10 percent per week. As you develop your training program and start to feel stronger, avoid the temptation to up your mileage or your weights too quickly. Remember that a diagnosis of overtraining syndrome could mean weeks or even months away from intense exercise.

Vary your training.

Periodize your training program by alternating hard and easy days, and varying training modalities. Muscle fibers and energy systems are stressed differently when performing sprints than when performing longer, slower workouts. After a hard workout, allow at least one to two days of lighter work or rest. Alternate cycling with in-line skating, or break up your running with swimming. Cross training improves fitness as it reduces risk of injury and overtraining.

Rest.

Rest at least one day a week, more if you are under extra stress or suspect that you are overdoing it. Rest gives your body the time it needs to rebuild and become stronger.

Cut back when needed.

Revise your training program when necessary, cutting back if you have symptoms of illness or overtraining. Cutting back now can save you weeks of recovery in the future.

Eat well.

Adequate fuel is essential for good performance. Endurance athletes should consume plenty of carbohydrates and some protein within two hours of workouts to ensure good energy stores for their next training session. Athletes attempting to lose weight while training are especially at risk for overtraining, since chronically low glycogen stores lead to fatigue and a decline in performance. A well-balanced diet also helps to prevent illness.

Drink plenty of fluids.

Adequate hydration helps to prevent fatigue and will keep you healthy.

Get adequate sleep and manage stress.

This may be the hardest recommendation of all. It's difficult to squeeze enough sleep, exercise, stress management and the rest of your life into each day. But stress can pile up and contribute to overtraining syndrome, so it's important to make time for recreation and relaxation.

The experts can hardly agree on recommendations for a minimal amount of exercise, although the range is about 30 to 60 minutes most days, and even up to 90 minutes if you are trying to lose weight. The definition of "too much exercise" is an even more complicated matter, and has to do with the effect exercise is having on your health and well-being. Getting too much exercise can be as harmful as getting too little exercise, since it can lead to long-term health problems and the disruptions in personal life that result from addiction and compulsive behavior.

For beginners: Don't do too much too soon.

Exercise professionals all agree that when starting a new exercise program, you must begin slowly and build gradually to avoid injury. It takes time for your body to adapt to the new demands you are placing on it. Cut back your exercise volume and intensity at the first sign of injury, and never increase training volume by more than 10 percent per week. If you have questions, a personal trainer or other fitness professional can help you get started. If you have health concerns, be sure to check with your health-care provider before you add to your exercise program.

Take at least one rest day a week, and balance exercise with recovery.

Peak performance results when you balance exercise with plenty of rest and good nutrition. Asking your body to do more than usual creates an overload. The overload stresses your body, and as your body recovers and adapts to the overload, you become stronger, more muscular, faster, or a better athlete in whatever capacities you are training.

Without rest, your body cannot adapt and performance suffers. So does your health. Symptoms of overtraining include the following:

- Decline in performance (e.g., you can't run your usual distance as fast as usual)
- Change in mood, increase in fatigue, irritability, depression, apathy
- Persistent aches and pains
- Elevation in resting heart rate
- More frequent incidents of cold and flu, symptomatic of a depressed immune response
- Trouble sleeping
- In women, disruption of the menstrual cycle
- Overuse injuries, such as stress fractures and tendonitis

You can balance training and recovery in several ways. Take at least one rest day each week. Athletes may take several days off before an important competition. A day off doesn't mean you must stay in bed. Just do something low intensity and different: walk on the beach, take your kids to the park or go for a swim. You can also increase performance and decrease risk of injury by alternating hard and easy days, and by cross training.

What if my goal is weight loss?

Your body still needs a day off every week to maintain health. And while experts recommend 60 to 90 minutes most days of the week to lose weight, you must begin slowly and build up to this level gradually. And like everyone else, you must cut back at the first sign of injury.

What if I am a competitive athlete in season?

Your coach has to train the whole team at one time, and training volume may be too high for you, especially early in the season. If you feel an injury coming on, see your athletic trainer right away. He will help the coach adjust your training schedule.

I need a lot of exercise to feel okay.

Regular physical activity reduces feelings of stress, anxiety and depression, and can be a great way to unwind and relax. It can also be fun! But when exercise becomes the only important thing in your life, interfering with your job, family, school or health, then exercise has become an unhealthy addiction. Other signs of exercise addiction include no longer experiencing pleasure during exercise, an inability to take a day off from exercise, and exercising when sick or injured.

Sometimes people with eating disorders use excessive exercise to purge calories and lose weight. Eating disorders such as anorexia nervosa and bulimia can quickly develop into dangerous health problems, causing irreparable damage to your bones, muscles and other organs, and to your metabolism. Eating disorders have the highest mortality rates of any psychiatric illness. If you feel like your eating and exercise habits have taken over your life, see your doctor for a referral to a specialist who can help you out of this dangerous situation.

27 Should Stretching Be a Part of Your Pre-Exercise Warm-Up?

Many serious athletes, recreational athletes, and weekend warriors have questions about whether to include or omit stretching from their warm-up routines. Several studies have raised questions about the benefits of pre-exercise stretching. Before making any changes in your warm-up routine, consider the following information.

Pre-exercise stretching may not be beneficial for everyone.

People who stretch during the pre-exercise warm-up generally do so because they believe that this practice will reduce risk of injury and muscle soreness. Studies suggest that for most sports, this may not be the case. When researchers have compared groups of people who stretch or don't stretch before activity, they have found little difference between the groups in rates of injury, types of injury, or muscle soreness. These observations have puzzled many researchers and fitness professionals.

While not all of the studies agree, they do indicate that we need more information on the physiology and biomechanics of stretching and flexibility. At this point, it appears that our intuition regarding the potential benefits of pre-exercise stretching do not have enough science to back them up. In fact, while pre-exercise stretching may be very beneficial for some sports and activities, it may be a waste of time for others, time that could be better spent in a more thorough warm-up.

In some cases, pre-exercise stretching may cause injury or interfere with athletic performance.

While most studies find neither benefit nor harm from pre-exercise stretching, the research is not unanimous. A few reports suggest slightly less injury in stretching groups, but others suggest *more* injury in those who stretch before exercise.

Studies have shown that stretching can increase muscle soreness and cause muscle damage. While such damage may be part of a process that promotes greater flexibility in the long run, just as muscle damage from strength training promotes stronger muscles in the long run, inducing such damage at the beginning of a workout does not make sense. In addition, improper stretching positions may cause harm to joints, by placing too much pressure on sensitive joint structures or by overstretching ligaments.

Another concern is that prolonged passive stretching appears to decrease a muscle's maximal force production. This can result in a decrease in strength for up to an hour after the stretch. This observation is of concern to athletes who participate in sports that require maximal muscle force production for performance, such as power lifting, basketball, football, soccer, volleyball, and many track and field events. Many runners and other endurance athletes have stopped stretching before exercise for this reason as well.

Given these concerns, it appears that stretching during the warm-up period may be a bad idea for some activities, especially those requiring strength and power. And it may be unnecessary in sports that do not require much flexibility.

Many people should still continue to include stretching in their warm-up routines.

If your sport or activity requires a great deal of flexibility, as is the case with gymnastics, dance, yoga, and some martial arts, you may still need to incorporate quite a bit of stretching into the warm-up to prepare for the upcoming activity.

Stretching is part of most physical therapy injury rehabilitation programs. If your therapist has advised special pre-exercise stretches, continue to follow these recommendations. And if stretching during the warm-up has kept you injury-free, remember that the research is not conclusive at this point. You may wish to continue stretching.

Everyone needs regular stretching for lifelong health and fitness.

If you decide that you don't need to stretch during your warm-up, you will still need to find another time to stretch, such as after exercise, or during a separate session. Stretching offers many health benefits. Flexibility, like all fitness measures, is governed by the "use it or lose it" rule. Although stretching before exercise does not appear to have very many short-term benefits, a lifetime of regular stretching can increase flexibility and slow the loss of flexibility that occurs as we age. Improvements in flexibility may also prevent back or other orthopedic problems in the future, and improve quality of life for older adults.

Motivational
Reading

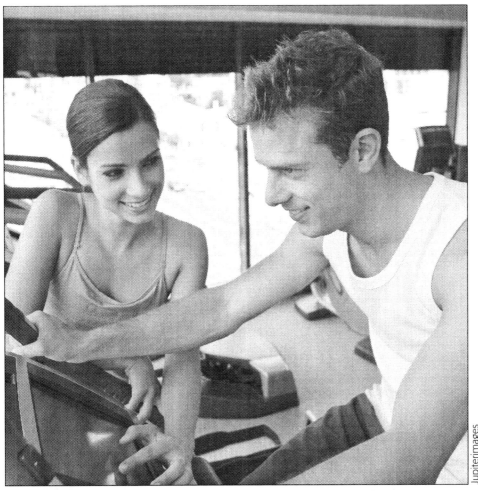

Jupiterimages

Chapter 3

Should You Make Time to Exercise?

If you are not currently very active, adding more exercise to your life may seem like a difficult thing to do. Exercise takes time and effort, and both of these often seem to be in short supply. And yet, you have heard that physical activity slows the aging process, helps prevent many of the chronic illnesses that run in your family, prevents weight gain, and helps you look and feel better. Many of your friends swear that regular exercise helps them feel less stressed, and more energetic. You wonder: could exercise help you?

A lack of activity is dangerous to your health.

Our bodies need plenty of movement to stay healthy. Without physical activity, bones, muscles, and joints weaken. Metabolism slows. Fat accumulates. Blood pressure rises, and blood sugar rises. Deposits grow on artery walls, reducing blood supply to the heart, brain, kidneys, and other vital organs. Studies estimate that being sedentary is as damaging to your health as being a smoker.

Unfortunately, physical activity has been engineered out of our daily lives. About the only common activities that count are heavy housework (such as washing windows and floors) and yard work (such as gardening and weeding), and most people do not perform these every day. Most of us have to create opportunities for more physical activity.

What's stopping you?

You are convinced of the benefits of regular physical activity, but you are having trouble getting started. Take some time to think about what's stopping you. Use your best problem-solving skills to brain storm some solutions. Almost everyone must rearrange their lives a bit when they wish to increase their level of physical activity.

Do you need more information? Be sure to check with your doctor if you are new to exercise and have any health concerns. Sometimes health-care providers can give you good information on exercising. Or you may wish to meet with a personal trainer. Community centers and fitness centers in your area may be able to refer you to someone.

Do you need more time? That is one of the most common problems. Is there a way to combine activity with your other responsibilities? Can you walk your errands or commute? When can you squeeze some exercise into your day? Maybe something else will have to go. What, nothing can go? Don't lose sight of the fact that your health is a priority. You are forced to make time for your health when you are sick; why not make time for it now, in order to avoid getting sick?

Form good intentions.

Making the decision to become more active is an important step. Reinforce your decision daily by reminding yourself of the benefits of regular physical activity. Read motivational books and articles. Talk to your friends who exercise. Find a friend who would like to join you. And take steps to prepare for your new schedule, and your new way of life.

Getting started: Preparation and planning increase fitness success.

What needs to be done now? You are ready to begin. Go ahead and sign up for that class, buy new walking shoes, or join that club. Call your friend and decide where and when to meet for your walk.

Review your exercise plans to be sure you are not biting off more than you can chew. Doing too much too soon is the leading cause of exercise injury. Start slowly and progress very gradually. Do everything you can to make your exercise safe. Use safety gear if you are going to bike or skate. Wear bright, reflective clothing if you will be walking or biking in traffic.

Spend some more problem-solving time anticipating problems that may come up, and plan strategies to keep moving. What will you do in bad weather? When it gets dark early? When there are disruptions at home or at work?

Realize that there are other things in your life besides your exercise program, and there will be times, no matter how hard you try (and you will try hard), that you will be unable to exercise. Resolve to keep these periods as brief as possible, and to return to your regular schedule as soon as you can. Remember that the greatest benefits come from regular, lifelong physical activity. A few weeks off won't matter…as long as you get right back into the routine.

Behavior Modification: Plan for Success

Rita and Margot enroll in an exercise class, both resolving to become lifelong exercisers. A year later, Rita is still exercising fairly regularly, while Margot does nothing more than take an occasional walk with friends. Why are some people more likely to stick with their resolutions than others?

Managing Stress and Coping With Negative Feelings

Stress is the number-one cause of exercise falling by the wayside. The ability to manage daily life stress protects people from the negative feelings that interfere with positive intentions. It takes energy to exercise regularly and eat in a new way. Stress causes negative feelings such as pressure, anxiety, depression, low self-esteem, fatigue, and anger. These feelings deplete our energy reserves, and make it more likely that we'll fall back into those comfortable old ways.

What's the best way to manage stress? Stress-management classes and workshops offer good advice on dealing effectively with sources of stress through better problem-solving, time-management, and communication skills. Cultivating a positive attitude and lifestyle that includes adequate sleep, a healthful diet and regular exercise helps as well. Many people find that regular physical activity provides the best antidote to stress.

If unhealthful habits have helped you deal with negative emotions, new methods of comforting yourself must be developed. Working out, talking to friends or doing something pleasurable like watching a funny movie can replace destructive coping methods like smoking or overeating.

Anticipating and Solving Problems

Problem-solving skills go hand in hand with stress management. Problems can easily disrupt newly established habits such as not smoking or skipping desserts. Problems often arise in the form of simple interruptions: visitors, parties, eating out and holidays. Anticipating and planning for these and more serious disruptions help to prevent that loss of control that accompanies a break from routine.

Sense of Control

People who persist in the face of difficulties often do so because they have a sense that what they do matters, that their decisions and actions can make a difference. People with this positive outlook are better problem-solvers and do not give up easily.

Supportive Environment

Supportive families, work places, communities and friends help the seeds of new habits take root. For example, a supportive workplace might offer flexible scheduling, access to exercise facilities or, at least, supervisors who won't look at you like you're crazy if you go for a walk during your lunch hour. Many exercisers find that the fitness center environment, along with its exercise instructors and personal trainers, provides support for a healthful lifestyle. Many support groups meet weekly to motivate people to sustain their progress. A personal trainer you check in with regularly serves the same purpose.

Self-Monitoring

People who successfully change lifestyle behaviors, such as exercise and eating habits, say that keeping track of their progress is especially helpful. Self-monitoring usually takes the form of a daily record of the behavior you are trying to change. People trying to establish an exercise habit can keep an exercise log. People trying to change their eating behaviors can write down what they eat each day.

Problematic Triggers

Certain factors stimulate a predictable response for each of us. For some people, walking into a bar for a beer means it's time to smoke a cigarette. Watching a movie might be a signal that triggers eating popcorn or candy. People who successfully change problematic behaviors try to identify signals that trigger these behaviors, and then work to change or eliminate the trigger situation, or at least plan more effective responses. For example, some people find it easier to quit smoking if they also quit drinking. If movies trigger too much junk food eating, switch to low-fat popcorn. If evening boredom triggers eating binges, get out of the house to attend interesting events.

Physical Activity

People who engage in regular physical activity are more likely to stick to their resolutions, even resolutions unrelated to exercise. Regular exercise helps reduce stress and gives a sense of control. Physical activity increases daily energy levels and provides a sense of personal well-being to sustain you through your challenging times.

Fitness Success: Working With Will Power

Changing a habit takes energy. Yet we tend to forget this when making resolutions to become more active. We often get carried away with our plans. It looks so easy on paper. But when we begin to translate our plans into daily life, we sometimes find that we cannot muster the will power required to overcome our old habits.

Will power refers to the control you exert over your thoughts, feelings, and behavior. Psychologists call this self-control. It takes self-control to change your routine. You use self-control when you roll out of bed in the morning and go for a walk, even though you would rather sleep another hour. But whatever you call it, will power, determination, or self-control, most people feel like they never have quite enough of it, especially when trying to start an exercise program.

Acknowledging that self-control is a limited resource can help you make more effective plans when it comes to increasing your level of physical activity. Working with your own level of self-control increases your likelihood of success. And understanding ways to reduce the amount self-control required by your exercise program means that your plans are more likely to succeed.

Acknowledge that daily exercise takes time and energy.

If you have exercised regularly before, you know that exercise can make you feel great, but that it does require time and energy. People most successful at sticking to their exercise programs admit that they really make an effort to do so, especially during the first six months. Assuming that adding exercise to your life will be easy almost guarantees failure. You must summon the energy to try hard, and persist in the face of the challenges that inevitably arise in daily life.

Increase your motivation to exercise by making your health a priority.

Motivation increases will power. How can you make your health a priority? Learn about how important exercise is to your health and well-being. People need at least 30 minutes of fairly vigorous physical activity most days of the week. Without activity, we are at greater risk of artery disease, obesity, high blood pressure, diabetes, and depression. How important is your health to you? Remember that an ounce of prevention is worth a pound of cure when it comes to chronic illness.

Exercise has immediate paybacks as well. Exercise reduces feelings of stress while it gives you energy. It improves sleep quality and mood. Look for these immediate rewards and remind yourself frequently of the importance of your long-term health.

Make physical activity a habit as quickly as possible.

Habits don't require self-control energy. Once exercise is part of your routine, you can operate on automatic pilot, and you may even feel disappointed if you must skip your exercise session for some reason. Habits develop most quickly when activity follows a "same time, same place" type of format. You may wish to do the same thing every day, or you might like some kind of weekly routine. You could, for example, walk Monday, Wednesday, and Saturday, and attend an exercise class Tuesday and Thursday. Set up a routine you will be most likely to follow. The more trouble you have had sticking to an exercise program, the more repetitious your routine should be. You want to avoid making decisions, which give you the opportunity to decide not to exercise!

Exercise with a friend.

Social support reduces the need for self-control. You can't decide not to exercise because your friend is waiting for you.

Exercise early in the day, if possible.

People who exercise first thing in the day have the best chance of sticking to their exercise programs. Self-control tends to be strongest at this time of day, and you are less likely to be derailed by other demands.

Exercise to reduce stress.

Stress is the leading cause of exercise program attrition. Coping with stress depletes your self-control energy. When you feel bad, doing something to help yourself feel better becomes more important than future health benefits. Learn to look to exercise to improve your mood and cope with stress.

Force of Habit:
Making Health and Fitness a Priority

If you have difficulty finding time to exercise, you are not alone. A perceived lack of time is one of the most common reasons that people fail to stick to their exercise programs. Even people with the best of intentions find themselves overwhelmed when tugged in too many directions at once. Somehow when others need you, self-care is the thing that gets put on hold.

Many busy people do manage to exercise regularly. How do they do it? By making their health and fitness a priority. One of the qualities that characterize success in any arena of life is an ability to take a long-range view of things, to see the total picture. Too often, we get caught up in short-term demands, and spend our time putting out fires at the expense of long-range strategic thinking and planning. This applies not only to the development of a healthful and satisfying lifestyle, but to every area of life, such as the development of meaningful careers and well-balanced families. The little things that have to get done somehow do get done, but the larger, really important issues can get put on hold indefinitely.

Make your health a priority before it becomes a necessity.

We take our health for granted until we get sick. People who swear they don't have a minute for self-care find themselves hospitalized for bypass surgery and out of commission for weeks. When our bodies force us to stay in bed, we do. We somehow manage to make the time when our health becomes that strong a priority.

But why wait? Think about your future, and all that you hope to do, in all the realms of your life. Isn't your health essential for the achievement of those goals? Unless you take care of your health, you cannot take care of business, family and other interests.

If not now, when?

If you are too busy to make exercise a priority now, when in the near future will you be less busy? Maybe you are lucky, and things will slow down in the next couple of weeks or months. But when most people ask themselves this question, they see the pace of their lives accelerating rather than slowing down, at least until retirement, or until children are grown and out of the house. If you are waiting for a better time to make exercise a priority, you may have to wait for too long.

Look for the benefits of regular physical activity.

When you look for the benefits of regular physical activity in your daily life, you reinforce the importance of fitness as a high-priority goal. After all, regular exercise is not only necessary to prevent chronic disease and disability; it also boosts your energy and helps you manage stress from day to day.

Enjoy the increased productivity that comes with good health. We're not just referring to the productivity of your work life, but to all parts of your life. When you are healthy and feeling good, you make better decisions and find more creative solutions to problems. You're more fun to be with and you have more to give to those you care about.

Employ the force of habit.

While any exercise is better than none, and it's never too late to benefit from an exercise program, the greatest benefits come from regular, vigorous, lifelong participation in physical activity. Irregular exercisers tend to encounter more frustration because they are constantly "starting over" and feeling out of shape. Since scheduling exercise is not part of their routine, the barriers to participation are greater.

People who manage to exercise regularly employ the force of habit. Exercise is a priority and part of their daily or weekly routine. Think about the busy people you know who still manage to exercise regularly. The people in their lives expect them to be unavailable at certain times and schedule accordingly. The most popular exercise time for the overbooked is first thing in the morning, before the rest of the world tries to derail you. But choose the times that work best for you.

Don't let the inevitable interruptions delay your speedy return.

While your fitness is a priority, interruptions in your exercise plan do occur. Injury, travel and piles of obligations may force you to give up some exercise time. Fortunately, in the context of a lifetime, a week or two with no exercise is no big deal, and you can congratulate yourself for your flexibility. But don't let a week or two off mean you take a year or two to get back to your program and reaffirm your commitment to exercise regularly.

How to Talk Yourself Into Regular Physical Activity

Do you ever talk yourself out of exercising? Have you ever caught yourself saying, "I'm too tired," "I'm too busy," or "I'll do it tomorrow?" If you tend to make excuses for skipping exercise, you can learn to overcome that little voice in your head that gets in the way of your commitment to take care of yourself. With practice, you can develop more positive ways of thinking that will support your efforts to engage in regular physical activity.

Examining Your Automatic Thoughts

As we grow from children into adults, we form certain patterns of thinking. Just as we develop lifestyle habits, such as brushing our teeth, we also develop habitual ways of perceiving the world. We can examine these automatic thoughts by listening to our self-talk, which is the way we talk to ourselves inside our minds.

For most people, self-talk includes not just talk, but also phrases, pictures, images, bits of songs and even complete sentences. It runs the gamut from *I can't believe it's Thursday already!* and *The chocolate one looks good,* to more emotionally laden images, such as being buried in work, or phrases like, *I'll never make it through this day.* Most of our self-talk is benign. But some automatic thoughts can be destructive when they reinforce negative beliefs and harmful behavior.

To uncover unproductive self-talk in the exercise department, simply observe your automatic thoughts for a week or two, and write down any thoughts that try to talk you out of exercising. Then take a look at your list. Which statements reflect real problems that need to be addressed? Brainstorm ways to deal with these problems. Which tend to be "excuses"? Is there a pattern? What are the common themes? Do certain phrases appear over and over?

Talking Back

To begin talking back to your negative self-talk, you must first take a look at the underlying beliefs that are causing the negative self-talk in the first place. Once you examine these underlying beliefs, you can form more positive and realistic self-talk that sounds convincing.

While many people know on one level that they need regular exercise to stay healthy, in their hearts there live other beliefs that conflict with their desire to stick to a program of regular physical activity. For example, some people may have been told as a child that sports were frivolous and that exercise was a waste of time. Others are perfectionists, and subconsciously believe that if they can't do something perfectly (for example, exercise every single day), then it's better to not do it at all. Many people (especially working parents) may believe it is wrong or selfish to take time out for themselves, when so many other people want more of their time. Some people worry that they look silly in exercise clothes, or that exercise is not appropriate for someone "their age."

Once you think about any mixed feelings you might have about exercise, you are ready to arm yourself with new self-talk to counteract that habitual self-talk that might pop into your mind just as you are preparing to enjoy your exercise session. Reformulate negative underlying beliefs, and construct new self-talk that reinforces your willingness to make your health a priority. For example, if you hear yourself thinking, "I'm too busy to exercise today. I'll do it tomorrow," argue back, "I am always busy, and tomorrow won't be much different. I'm still going to take my lunch hour to get to the gym. The exercise will give me energy and help me get more done this afternoon." To counteract, "Exercise is a waste of time," try thinking, "I need regular exercise to stay healthy and manage stress. What is more important than my health? I must take care of my health so that I can do my work and take care of my family."

You might also wish to use these new statements as a kind of internal cheerleading to help you stick to your exercise program.

Stick to Your Exercise Program: Find an Exercise Partner

Some people seem to work exercise seamlessly into their days. No matter what happens, they manage to make it to the gym, or go out for a jog. But some of us have more trouble following through on our plans to become more active. Life gets in the way and there are so many other things that need our attention.

We know that exercise helps keep us healthy, and that our health is a priority. But that knowledge alone is not enough to get us moving. If this sounds like you, then making a commitment to an exercise partner might be just the thing to get you out the door.

Why Are Exercise Partners Helpful?

Exercise partners provide gentle coercion that helps you stick to your exercise program. Many people are more likely to do something if someone else is counting on them. If someone is waiting for you, you have no opportunity to talk yourself out of exercise.

Good exercise partners also help to make fitness fun. Friendly company helps to change the channel on a stressful day. And conversation helps to pass the time, if you find exercise boring.

Factors to Consider When Choosing an Exercise Partner

If you think some company might help you stick to your exercise program, why not invite someone to exercise with you? The most important consideration when deciding who to ask is compatibility. You want to be with someone whose company you enjoy, and who can keep up with you.

In addition to compatibility, you will need to find someone who might enjoy the activities you are doing. Walking and jogging are easy to do with someone else if you like the same pace. Some exercise partners work out together at a fitness center. They may exercise on adjacent machines that allow for conversation, or they may separate during their workouts, but stretch together at the end. Sometimes exercise partners attend the same group exercise class. Even though they do not talk to each other during class, they have a chance to catch up before and after the class. And they make sure the other person gets to class each time.

Scheduling can be a major hurdle. You'll need to find a partner whose schedule allows him or her to join you when you are also free. Be sure your exercise plans are as convenient as possible. If exercising with a partner makes exercise less convenient or more time consuming, you'll have more excuses than ever to drop out of your exercise program. Remember, a partner should make exercise easier, not harder.

Be Creative as You Think About Exercise Partners

An exercise partner need not be your best friend. Consider coworkers, or members of groups you belong to. Is there someone from your book club, parent group, weight control group, church or synagogue you might like to spend time with? Perhaps a friendship will blossom as you get to know each other better!

Is there someone you should be spending more time with? At work, you may be able to turn a meeting into a walk. Since you won't want to carry your laptop, or paper and pen, walking is most conducive to reporting-type meetings that don't require note taking.

What about family members? You may be able to find an activity that allows you to spend time with your spouse. Parents may wish to use activity time as quality time with a child or teen. Some parents report that they get more conversation out of their sons and daughters when they are doing something active together than when they ask at dinnertime, "How was school?" Shared activity can be a way to strengthen these important relationships.

Dogs provide a wonderful exercise opportunity. Spend more time walking your dog, if you have one. You and your dog both need exercise to stay healthy!

Plan for Days When Your Partner is Unavailable

Exercise may be more fun with a partner, but don't let lack of a partner keep you from exercising. When your partner calls in sick, be ready with a backup plan. Take a walk alone, or listen to a book on tape when you work out at the fitness center. If you like to be with people but lose your exercise partner, sign up for a group exercise class and join in the fun.

Fitness Motivation: What Moves You to Move?

You know you should be physically active almost every day to stay healthy. But you have probably also noticed that knowing what you should do and actually doing it are two different things. Fitting fitness into your everyday life can be a challenge. How do you find the motivation to be active when time and energy feel like they are in short supply?

Making the Decision to Become More Active

Motivation often evolves from a decision to begin an exercise program, or to increase your level of activity. Sometimes people suddenly decide now is the time to start an exercise program, but more often they spend some time thinking about the costs and benefits of starting or changing their exercise habits. It may take considerable thought and planning before you are ready to make a commitment to lifestyle change.

Many factors may motivate decisions to become more active. Behavior change can be difficult, so sometimes people resist change until they become uncomfortable with the way things are. For example, people often carry a vague intention to exercise more that never turns into a solid decision to exercise until they are faced with a medical diagnosis, such as type 2 diabetes, that requires physical activity as a component of treatment. The discomfort from receiving such a diagnosis is relieved by the decision to begin exercising.

Some people are motivated by a concern for family or friends. For example, they may decide to begin exercising to provide good self-care role models for their children, or start walking with a friend or spouse who needs support to get out the door.

Many people decide to become more active only after major consciousness-raising changes in their self-evaluation, and changes in their habitual assumptions and thought patterns. While most people will say that exercise is important, they may not really feel this in their hearts. But situations may arise that remind them that it is important to put their health first for perhaps an hour each day, which prompts a decision to exercise. Such shifts in self-evaluation may occur not only in response to health problems, but also in response to other stressful life situations.

What Motivates People to Implement a Decision to Exercise?

Making the decision to exercise is not nearly as hard as sustaining a commitment to be more active. But that decision may contain ideas that can provide continuing motivation for you. Remind yourself daily of the important reasons you decided to become more active, and use these reasons to fan the flames of your desire to be fitter, healthier, less stressed, or whatever has gotten you started.

Positive Versus Negative Reasons for Exercise

Some research suggests that people who express positive reasons for exercising are more likely to stick to their exercise programs than people who voice negative reasons for exercising. Positive reasons include things such as exercising to feel more energetic, to have fun, to get stronger, or become healthier. Negative reasons include exercising to lose weight or improve appearance, especially when these reasons evolve from feelings of inadequacy or low self-esteem.

Sometimes positive and negative reasons are two sides of the same coin. A person who needs to lose weight may be more motivated by deciding to exercise to feel healthier, rather than simply focusing on weight loss. Weight loss is often considered a negative reason not because it is a "bad" reason, but because weight loss occurs fairly slowly (when it is fat loss), and exercisers may get frustrated that results take too long.

Intrinsic Versus Extrinsic Motivation

Psychologists tell us that people with intrinsic motivation to exercise tend to exercise more regularly than those with extrinsic motivation. Intrinsic motivation means you exercise for reasons connected to the exercise experience itself. You may love a competitive tennis match, need to walk to work, enjoy bicycling, or relish the break from work provided by a workout at the fitness center. Extrinsic motivation occurs when you exercise because the doctor or someone else told you to, or you want to earn points for a free t-shirt.

Most people have a combination of intrinsic and extrinsic motivations for exercise. If you have decided to exercise in response to doctor's orders, try to feel that making time for self-care is an important responsibility to yourself and to those you love. Take charge of your exercise program so that it includes activities you enjoy the most (or hate the least!) and is as convenient as possible.

Positive Reinforcement

Look for positive results from exercise. When you find that exercise improves sleep quality, reduces stress, gives you energy, or becomes time to spend with friends, your motivation to exercise grows stronger.

More Than an Exercise Program

Have you ever noticed that when you have to do something, you don't want to do it as much as the things you choose to do? This may explain why people who view their exercise activities as an opportunity to have fun, be with a friend or manage stress tend to exercise more regularly than people who see exercise as a painful or boring obligation. When you see physical activity as beneficial in your daily life, perhaps even as an opportunity for recreation, exercise looks more appealing. If you would like physical activity to provide more than physical fitness, think about whether you would like to incorporate any of the factors below into your exercise program.

Time With Family or Friends

Are there family members or friends you would like to spend more time with? You could talk as you walk together, or participate in another activity that you would both enjoy.

Group Support

The energy of a group exercise class or a sports team can help you work harder or have more fun than exercising alone.

Time Alone

Some people need a break from other people and find that break with exercise. They may enjoy a solitary workout or being alone in a crowd. A repetitive activity such as walking can provide an opportunity for problem solving and creative thinking.

Time Outdoors

Sunlight and fresh air are therapeutic, especially for people who spend most of their time indoors. Consider walking, hiking, bicycling or skating. If there's snow, try skiing (downhill or cross-country), snowshoeing or sledding.

Opportunity for Concentration or Competition

Some people enjoy activities that force them to take a mental break from daily life. Competitive sports such as tennis, racquetball and golf, and adventure activities that require concentration, such as whitewater kayaking and rock climbing, force problems out of your mind. If these appeal to you, investigate opportunities in your area. Many masters programs exist for various sports.

Meditation

In disciplines such as yoga and tai chi, you strive for emotional balance through activity, deep breathing and a meditative focus. These activities are usually appropriate for a wide range of fitness levels and ages, and many people find them a nice change of pace. Repetitive activities such as walking, running, cycling and swimming can also provide opportunities for rhythmic breathing and a meditative mental state.

Purpose

Do you like to feel you have accomplished something with your activity? People who successfully incorporate physical activity into their lives year after year often do so because the chosen activity has a purpose. People may walk or bike for transportation, or garden in order to have beautiful flowers or fresh vegetables.

Fun

When you were a kid, you probably were active because you enjoyed playing games, riding your bike and doing other activities with your friends. Nothing beats having a good time. You can add fun to exercise in many simple ways. Watch funny movies when you work out, go dancing or plan an active vacation.

Meaning

Many people use physical activity to create meaning in their lives. For example, many people enjoy connecting with nature while hiking or performing other outdoor activities. Others train for events that involve fundraising for personally meaningful charities. Physical activity may provide a vehicle for strengthening relationships among family and friends. Mind/body activities may involve a search for emotional balance and philosophical understanding.

Quality of Life

As you expand the ways that physical activity can enrich your life, you will become aware of the many emotional health benefits of exercise. You may feel more energetic and less fatigued, irritable and stressed. These psychological benefits strengthen exercise's physical health benefits, and enhance the quality of your daily life. As many people have observed, physical activity will not only add years to your life, but life to your years!

36 Imaginative Planning Helps Overcome Barriers to Exercise

Regular physical activity gives you enormous health benefits. But to develop these health benefits, you must participate in almost daily physical activity for the rest of your life.

Sound impossible? Fortunately, the rest of your life unfolds one day at a time, and within each day there are opportunities for physical activity. The trick is to find or create such opportunities. If you tend to let life get in the way of your exercise program, read on. A little positive visualization can help you turn your exercise intentions into healthful physical activity.

Good Intentions

The road to health is paved with good intentions. But as everyone knows, good intentions alone are not enough, especially when it comes to exercise. These intentions must be translated into daily physical activity.

Most people have a good plan of action when they first begin an exercise program. They have some sort of workout schedule, and they follow it for a while. But as time goes by, complications inevitably arise. Other obligations compete for that exercise time, and before long, weeks have elapsed, and it's difficult to get back into the exercise habit.

Renewing your commitment to good health with a few minutes of visualization each day can reinforce your exercise habit. Visualization enables you to harness the power of your imagination to help solve the problems that get in the way of your exercise commitment, and to manage the stress that can interfere with your good intentions.

Focus on the Process

Most people have very active imaginations. Here's how to put yours to good use: Pick a time during the day when you can spend a few minutes relaxing. Many people find that first thing in the morning is best. Others prefer the end of the day, or some other quiet time. Take a few deep breaths and bring your awareness to the present moment, undistracted by your daily list of Things to Do. Focus on your breathing and feel your muscles relax.

Imagine yourself getting to your exercise class, going for a walk, or whatever you have planned for physical activity that day. What will you be doing before your exercise time? How will you leave that activity? What happens next? Try to make the scene as vivid as possible. As you begin to imagine your transition into physical activity, you might become aware of problems that may arise. Take a moment to think about these. How might you best deal with them? If you will be unable to go forward with your original exercise plan, what are some alternatives? Is there a later class you can take? Can you walk earlier in the day? Let your imagination come up with some creative solutions for any barriers that might arise. If you must miss your exercise session that day, plan for your return the next day, or as soon as possible.

Be aware of how you are feeling as you imagine these scenes. Using your imagination in this way helps you to practice coping with negative feelings that might weaken your resolve to exercise. Recognize that negative feelings are a part of life, and that, in fact, exercise can help you reduce feelings of anger, frustration and fatigue.

Remind yourself of the rewards of physical activity, and the reasons you decided to start exercising in the first place. Remember how good you feel after your workout. Remember that your health is a priority. Without your good health, your other commitments will suffer. Once you have practiced this visualization exercise a few times, it may take as little as 10 minutes a day.

Not to Worry

Be sure your visualization practice does not degenerate into fruitless or stressful worrying. If you are coping with depression or other stress disorders, visualizing difficult situations may only make matters worse. Check with your health-care provider if you need help for depression or for coping with a difficult situation.

Think Positive and Stick to Your Exercise Program

I'm too fat. I'm too out of shape. I've really gone downhill this past year. These negative thoughts sometimes provide helpful motivation for beginning an exercise program. But research shows that people who turn exercise into a punishment that reinforces low self-esteem are more likely to drop out of an exercise program than their friends who make exercise an enjoyable experience that helps them feel good about themselves.

Find positive reasons to exercise.

Everyone needs plenty of daily physical activity to feel good and to prevent chronic illness. People who exercise because they want to stay healthy, or to overcome certain health limitations, have more success sticking to their exercise programs. This may be because they are more likely to see the progress they are looking for compared to people who expect dramatic changes in appearance, such as unrealistic weight loss.

If your primary goal is weight loss, be sure you are trying to lose weight for positive reasons—to improve your health, to reduce your risk of chronic illness and to feel good. Focus on improving your fitness, and cultivating healthful eating and exercise habits that you can maintain for years to come. Exercise because you want to make the most of who you are, and so that you can live a fulfilling, productive life.

Other positive reasons for exercise include wanting to reduce feelings of stress, have more energy, spend time with friends, get outdoors and have fun. Some people exercise because they enjoy the competition and camaraderie of playing sports, or because they enjoy the challenge of working to meet a fitness or performance goal.

Be sure your exercise program matches your health and fitness goals.

It's easier to stick to your exercise program when you feel it is helping you make progress toward your health and fitness goals. Think about what you would like to accomplish with your exercise program, then decide what types of activities would help you reach those goals. If you need help figuring this out, speak with an exercise instructor or personal trainer.

Make exercise a positive experience.

Make your exercise program as convenient and enjoyable as possible – one that fits into your lifestyle. Find a time of day that works for you, and activities that you like. A good exercise program should help you feel invigorated and refreshed after your workout. Get a friend or family member to join you!

Find a comfortable exercise environment.

When looking for a fitness center, convenience will probably be your primary consideration. In addition, look for friendly staff members who make you feel welcome. Most fitness centers are a little intimidating until you have been there a few times, so don't expect to feel immediately "at home." However, if the center feels too unwelcoming, you may have difficulty sticking to your exercise plans.

If you tend to worry about your appearance, avoid exercising in front of mirrors. You want exercise to help you feel better, not worse! If your reflection detracts from a positive exercise experience in a group exercise setting, try to stand on the side of the class, or behind another student who blocks your view of the mirror (not the instructor). Remind yourself that some mirrors make you look larger than you really are. Focus on your workout, not on your reflection.

Find exercise clothes that make you feel good. Choose apparel that feels comfortable, looks good on you and makes movement a pleasure.

Consider strength training.

Consider adding strength training to your exercise program. Many fitness centers offer strength-training classes for beginners. Some places offer classes especially for older adults or for people with specific health limitations, such as arthritis or back problems.

Many people report health and fitness benefits after only a few months of regular strength training. Just two or three sessions a week can lead to noticeable improvements in strength, muscle tone, posture, and self-esteem.

38 The Pleasure Principle

What images come to mind when you think of a healthful lifestyle? An emaciated macrobiotics devotee munching on nuts and twigs? Your aerobics instructor who exercises at least three hours a day? The lean and mean marathoner you see pounding the pavement on your way to work every day? A health spa lifestyle where activity is devoted to helping you look and feel good? Slender, young magazine models?

Several things are wrong with these images. Some are turn-offs: They make a healthful lifestyle look like a prison sentence. If a low-fat diet means plain dry toast every day, who needs it? If exercise is seen as uncomfortable, bothersome, burdensome or humiliating, why not do as W.C. Fields suggested: Whenever you feel the urge to exercise, lie down until it goes away.

Some healthy lifestyle images are attractive, even inspirational, but unobtainable for most of us. When we compare ourselves to them, the disparity is too discouraging. We'll never get there. We feel frustrated with our feeble attempts and throw in the towel. We develop an all-or-nothing attitude: If I can't lose 10 pounds in two weeks, I might as well not bother to try. If my muscle definition hasn't improved noticeably by the end of the month, I'll quit this nonsense.

New Attitude

A good attitude is the cornerstone of a healthful lifestyle for several reasons. First of all, a healthful lifestyle will have much better health promotion value if you enjoy it. Worrying too much about what you eat or whether you are following the best exercise program is harmful to your health. Becoming self-absorbed and obsessed with your risk factors significantly decreases the benefits you would otherwise accrue from your healthful lifestyle program. In fact, research is beginning to show that cultivating an optimistic, positive outlook is an important heart-health risk reducer, while hostility, cynicism, alienation, self-absorption, and loneliness are the Type-A characteristics that increase your risk of heart disease. Lifestyle change without this positive attitude means you are missing important pieces of the health-promotion puzzle.

Be Real

Unrealistic ideas about how to achieve a healthful lifestyle are self-defeating because they set you up for failure. You can never do enough or achieve enough. Successful exercise programs are ones that are feasible. They are realistic in terms of time commitment, accessibility and cost. Most of all they fit into your lifestyle.

Dietary changes must fit, as well. Many of us know people who are either "on" or "off" a diet. Very restrictive diets are an unnatural way of eating, based on monotony and self-denial. They are difficult to live with, and people following such diets often experience frustration, fatigue, depression, low self-esteem and uncontrollable food cravings. They go off the diet and over-indulge in the "forbidden" foods. The stress created by restrictive diets is worse for your health than being somewhat overweight and enjoying your food.

That is not to say you should throw caution to the wind and indulge your way to a heart attack. There is no denying that good nutrition, not smoking, and moderate exercise are connected to good health. But the way we respond to this connection can be the difference between a healthy desire to take good care of ourselves and an unhealthy obsession with following the "perfectly correct" lifestyle.

Enjoy!

Feeling good is the opposite of feeling stressed. While chronic excess stress and negative emotions lead to harmful physiological changes, positive emotions create health. Pleasure and positive emotions are often associated with a relaxed contentment and feeling of well-being. Such feelings activate the relaxation response, a physiological state characterized by lower heart rate, blood pressure and breathing rate, and muscle relaxation, lower levels of stress hormones, and improved immune response. While a chronic stress response leads to an assortment of negative health effects, a frequent relaxation response helps prevent these ills because it tugs your body in the other direction. Positive emotions also seem to have an effect beyond the relaxation response, and lead to healthful physical changes. Besides, if something like your exercise program makes you feel good, you will want to keep doing it—for the rest of your life.

Nutrition and Health

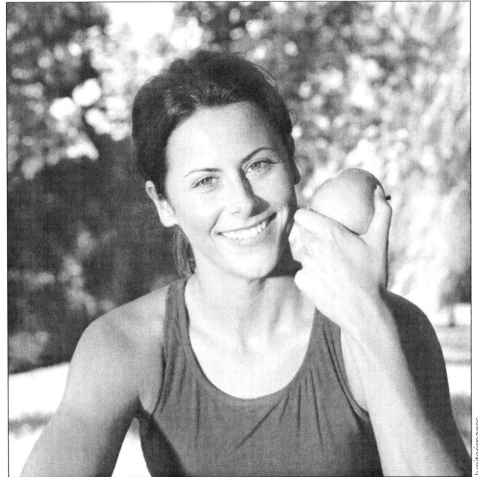

Jupiterimages

Chapter 4

Nutrition 101: Eating for Good Health

Most health-minded consumers are well acquainted with the food pyramid and the basic food groups. The food pyramid provides guidelines for healthy eating, but only if you make good choices within each food group. People eating to prevent or reverse artery disease, and anyone concerned about weight control, will want to be especially careful to limit empty calories, as well as foods high in harmful fats. Following are a few basic guidelines for making healthy choices.

Choose whole-grain foods, especially those high in fiber.

Carbohydrates, including those found in grains, cereal, pasta and baked goods, provide ready energy. Best choices are high in fiber and low in added fats, especially saturated fats, and sugars. Try whole-grain cereals and breads. Brown rice and products prepared from whole grains, such as tabouleh, are available in many grocery stores and restaurants.

Eat plenty of fruits and vegetables.

Shoot for the high end of recommended servings for fruits and vegetables, which are about three to five servings of vegetables and two to four servings of fruits. Don't worry if you eat more, as long as your choices consist mostly of fruits and vegetables without added sugars or sauces that are high in saturated fats (such as butter or cheese sauces). Choose baked potatoes over French fries. Fruits contain more fiber and nutrients than fruit juices. Avocados and olives have heart-healthy fat and can be included in a heart-healthy diet in moderation.

Look for low- and non-fat dairy products.

Whole milk, cream, and their products are high in saturated fat, which increases risk for heart disease. If you do not consume dairy products, be sure to include other sources of calcium, vitamin D, and magnesium in your diet.

Go for variety in the protein group.

Limit protein selections that are high in saturated fats, such as high-fat meats and poultry, but freely include high-fat fish, such as salmon, since this type of fat reduces heart disease risk. Many health experts advise eating fish once or twice a week. The same advice applies to nuts and seeds, such as walnuts, almonds, sunflower and sesame seeds, etc. Since these foods are relatively high in calories, they need to replace other foods, such as meat; simply adding these foods to your diet may result in weight gain. Legumes (beans) are high in protein, fiber, and many vitamins and minerals, and have no fat. Try lentil or other bean soups, and add beans to your salads and casseroles.

Reduce intake of foods high in saturated and trans fats.

Foods high in saturated fats are commonly found in the milk and meat groups, although certain plant oils, such as coconut and palm oil, are also high in saturated fat. In the milk group, look for skim milk and nonfat dairy products, such as nonfat yogurt and nonfat cottage cheese. Small amounts of regular cheese and low-fat cheese can be used for flavoring, such as small portions of cheese crumbled onto a salad.

Trans fats are found in any product containing hydrogenated oils, especially some margarine, some peanut butter, salad dressing and baked goods. Trans fats have the same negative health effects as saturated fats and should be kept to a minimum in the diet.

Healthy fats can be included in your diet.

Choose healthful sources of dietary fat—nuts and seeds, avocados, plant oils, such as olive and flaxseed oil, and fish. These foods contain fatty acids that are essential for good health. In moderation, these fats also reduce heart disease risk.

Get regular physical activity.

Try to get at least 30 minutes of moderately vigorous physical activity each day. Balance calorie intake with exercise to maintain a healthy weight.

Sport Nutrition for Peak Performance

Good nutrition is important for everyone, especially for athletes who have rigorous training and performance schedules. Food provides the fuel and chemicals our bodies need to produce energy and maintain good health. While many nutrition basics apply to everyone, athletes do have some special requirements.

Water

Water is vital for health and performance. Endurance athletes should drink plenty of water throughout the day, and about a half-cup for each 15 to 20 minutes of exercise. After exercise, drink about 2 cups of fluids for every pound of weight lost.

Calories

Physical activity requires energy, and lots of it. Your diet must supply the raw materials that your body needs to maintain a high-energy output and to rebuild energy stores. Your body gets energy from carbohydrates, protein and fat. In general, athletes should try to get at least 60 percent of their calories from carbohydrates, about 15 percent from protein and about 25 percent from fat.

How do you know if you are getting enough calories? In general, you are probably getting enough if you are not gaining or losing weight, and if you have plenty of energy to meet your training and performance needs. Adolescent athletes have especially high-energy needs, since they need extra energy for growth and development, in addition to the energy requirements of physical activity. Irregular menstrual cycles in women may indicate insufficient caloric intake.

Carbohydrates

During physical activity, your body relies primarily on a form of carbohydrate called glycogen, which is stored in the liver and muscles. Glycogen is quickly broken down into glucose, which is then used to make energy. When glycogen stores are low, you will tire more quickly and your performance will decline. Your body makes glycogen from the carbohydrates that you eat.

Consume carbohydrate sources such as fruits, vegetables and whole grains that contain vitamins and minerals. Glycogen is resynthesized most quickly during the first two hours after exercise, so consuming a high-carbohydrate drink or snack after exercise helps your glycogen stores get ready for your next workout or performance.

Protein

Athletes require somewhat more protein than less-active people. This is because some protein is burned for energy during endurance activities and is made into muscle in response to the demands of strength training. The usual protein requirement for healthy adults is about 0.4 grams of protein per pound of body weight per day. People who are considerably overweight should estimate protein requirements based on what they should weigh, since extra fat weight does not require increased protein intake. Endurance athletes need about 0.5 to 0.6 grams per pound per day, while strength athletes may need as much as 0.6 to 0.7 grams.

Protein is most likely to be used for fuel if carbohydrate intake is too low, so consuming plenty of carbohydrates helps to protect protein stores. Look for low-fat protein sources; people who exercise and play sports should still consume a heart-healthy diet.

Vitamins and Minerals

Athletes require somewhat higher levels of B vitamins. The increased caloric intake that accompanies training usually provides adequate levels of these vitamins. A multivitamin supplement that contains 100 percent of the daily vitamin requirements is an alternative for athletes whose diets fall short.

Many athletes try to consume plenty of fruits and vegetables to ensure a good supply of chemicals called antioxidants. During exercise, oxygen consumption increases dramatically, creating chemicals called free radicals, which are natural byproducts of aerobic metabolism. Antioxidants help to limit the damage caused by free radicals. A good variety of fruits and vegetables contain these helpful chemicals. These sources also supply many of the minerals that are important for physical activity, including chromium, magnesium and potassium.

Iron deficiency sometimes occurs in athletes. Since iron supplements are thought to increase oxidative damage, it's important to avoid them unless your doctor has diagnosed you with iron-deficiency anemia and recommends them. Zinc, found in meat, eggs, seafood and whole-wheat products, is important in energy metabolism and is also sometimes low in athletes' diets.

Optimal Hydration for Peak Performance

Physical activity increases your fluid needs in several ways. You sweat during exercise to get rid of excess heat. You also lose water when you breathe, especially when the air is dry, since you humidify the air in your lungs. Cold air holds little moisture, and you can lose over a liter of fluid when you exercise for several hours in the winter.

In cold air or water, your blood huddles into your core to prevent heat loss. But this change in core blood volume stimulates the kidneys to make urine, another form of fluid loss. As you warm up and circulation expands back into the skin, this water needs to be replaced for optimal performance.

It's easy to keep up with your increased fluid needs if you keep an eye on your water intake. While thirst tells you it's time to drink, athletes need to drink before the thirst mechanism is activated in order to keep up with rapid fluid losses during exercise, especially when exercise is vigorous and lasts over 30 minutes. The following are some guidelines to help you be sure you are getting enough to drink.

Weigh yourself before and after physical activity.

Weight loss is a good indicator of dehydration. Each pound of lost weight means you should have drunk another 2 cups of fluids before and during exercise. If you practice weighing yourself before and after exercise you can calculate your water deficit.

Check the color of your urine throughout the day.

Urine should be pale in color. Dark, concentrated urine indicates dehydration. Some vitamin supplements cause deep yellow urine. If this is your case, then monitor urine volume, which should be plentiful.

Practice drinking adequate fluids during training.

Learning how to stay hydrated is especially important if you are training for an event requiring prolonged, vigorous activity, such as a marathon or triathlon. Part of your training is to figure out how much water you typically lose for a given period of time under standard conditions (whatever they are for your area), and then practice staying hydrated.

If you will be consuming sports drinks, figure out which sports drinks work best for you during your training workouts, not on race day! Some people find certain drinks, especially those containing fructose, cause abdominal cramps or diarrhea when consumed during vigorous exercise.

Drink plenty of water before an important competition.

You are limited in how much water you can absorb during exercise, so it is possible to lose water more quickly than you can replace it. Therefore, it is important to begin your long workout or contest well hydrated. Drink plenty of fluids during the 24 hours preceding your event. Then drink two or three cups of water or a sports drink two or three hours before the event. Finally, drink another cup 10 or 20 minutes before the race begins.

Drink during exercise.

You figured out how much water you typically need to replace and how much you could comfortably drink during your training, remember? Optimal water intake during a contest varies widely, but sports nutritionists generally recommend about a cup every 15 minutes, more if you are larger or a heavy sweater. Water is fine for shorter (less than one hour) events. If you will be exercising longer, a sports drink might be helpful to keep your blood sugar levels up and replace electrolytes (especially sodium and potassium) lost in sweat.

But do not drink too much.

Sodium levels in the blood can dip too low when sodium losses through sweating are combined with excessive water intake. Most cases occur in slow, inexperienced marathoners (over four hours) who exercise at lower intensities and drink too much water.

Drink after exercise.

If your workout or event was quite long, you may not have been able to drink enough to keep up with fluid losses. Drink two cups of fluids for every pound of weight lost. Sports drinks are especially helpful if you have become dehydrated. Consuming fluids with carbohydrate soon after exercise will help your body replenish glycogen stores.

Carbohydrate Loading: Avoiding a Fuel Shortage

If you have ever run out of energy during exercise you know how bad it feels. Your legs turn to lead and it takes all the willpower in the world to keep them moving. Your head swims and you turn into somebody else, exhausted, dizzy, heart pounding, moving in slow motion, as in a dream.

For thousands of years, athletes have experimented with their diets in attempts to improve fuel availability and performance. Once exercise scientists understood that glycogen supplied the best fuel for prolonged high intensity exercise, they began to investigate ways to pack more glycogen into the muscles and liver with the goal of helping endurance athletes avoid a fuel shortage during training and contests. Many athletes whose events last longer than 90 minutes practice some form of carbohydrate loading before an important contest to maximize their glycogen stores.

Does carbohydrate loading really improve performance?

Athletes vary greatly in their individual responses to carbohydrate loading. Some athletes find it very helpful, while others don't see much improvement in their performance. Changing your diet before a big race can also have disastrous effects. If the foods don't agree with you, you may end up with abdominal cramps or diarrhea, which can really slow you down. Be sure to try out any dietary changes before one of your training days, not before race day.

I have heard carbohydrate loading is less effective in women. Is this true?

In general, women seem to increase muscle glycogen stores to a lesser extent than men in response to carbohydrate loading, but again the results vary enormously from person to person. Studies suggest that women do benefit from adding some carbohydrate calories to their diets for several days before a contest.

What's the best way to increase glycogen stores?

The first step to increasing muscle glycogen stores is exercise training. Endurance athletes exercise hard to get not only their heart and muscles in shape, but also to train their energy production systems to crank out ATP from fuel and oxygen. Their muscles get better at storing glycogen for energy, and turning it into glucose for quick fueling.

An important part of training is learning how to eat. You will need to cultivate good eating habits that support your exercise habit. In general, you want to eat a balanced diet, with plenty of fruits, vegetables, whole grains, and legumes. These carbohydrate foods provide not only energy but also fiber, vitamins, and minerals. Adequate protein, healthful fats, and water are also important.

Learn which foods your digestive system can accommodate in your pre-race "meal," probably more of a snack, a few hours before the competition. Get in the habit of replenishing glycogen following workouts, consuming some carbohydrate drinks or snacks within one hour of a workout.

Beginning two or three weeks before the big event, begin to taper your workouts. While hard training makes you stronger, it does so by stressing your body. Giving your body extra recovery time not only maximizes glycogen storage, but also allows your muscles to completely heal, and you to compete at your strongest.

Three days before the event, trade in some of your fat calories for carbohydrates. Since you have tapered your training and are burning fewer calories during the day, you probably do not need to add calories to your diet. (The exceptions are athletes, especially females, who restrict calories somewhat during training.) Carbohydrates should make up at least 65 percent of your calories, and you should consume at least 4 grams of carbohydrate per pound of body weight (8 grams/kg).

You will know your glycogen stores are packed if you gain 2 to 4 pounds by race day. This is mostly water weight, because each gram of carbohydrate is stored with 3 grams of water, which will also come in handy during an endurance event.

Eating Well for Less

Rising food and energy costs are becoming a fact of life. Unless your income rises as quickly as prices, something has to go. Many people are taking a close look at their spending habits, including the money they spend on food.

Trimming food costs can be tricky, because you don't want to sacrifice your long-term health in the process. Value meals at fast food restaurants may supply a lot of calories, but may also supply a lot of fat, salt, and sugar. Cheap in the short run may be expensive later, if you develop nutrition-related illnesses such as diabetes, cardiovascular disease, or cancer. How can you reduce food expenditures and yet maintain a healthful diet?

Evaluate your eating and spending habits.

Make some time to think about your weekly routine, if you have one. If you are in charge of food for your family, include your family's habits. You might keep a food diary for a few days, noting what you ate, where you bought it, and what it cost.

Once you have a good idea of your eating habits, think about which habits promote good nutrition. In general, the best diets have an abundance of vegetables and fruits each day (five to nine servings), lean protein sources (meat, fish, poultry, beans, eggs), low-fat dairy foods, and whole grains. You can improve your diet by reducing your consumption of foods high in added fats and sugars.

Organize and plan.

Improving your eating and spending habits requires you to be more intentional about your eating behavior at first. It takes some time and energy to make good nutrition a priority. What are two or three changes you could make in your eating and spending habits that would lead to the most improvements, in nutrition, your budget, and quality of life?

Start with changes that won't feel too stressful. For example, you might eat better for less by taking your lunch to work. If you can't face preparing a lunch every day (or every evening), try planning ahead for just two or three days. Eventually these changes become habits that require less energy and forethought.

Reduce junk eating and spending.

Are there opportunities to reduce empty calorie (low nutrition) snack foods and beverages? You do not need to eliminate every treat, but start with the convenience foods you grab when you are hungry and busy, things high in fats

and sugars you may not necessarily really enjoy. What will you eat instead?

Prepare your own snacks and beverages for when you are away from home.

Reach for the fruit, yogurt, nuts, and other healthful snack foods you take along. Keep them in portion-sized containers to avoid overeating. And just take along as much as you want to eat for the day. The same goes for beverages. Make your own coffee drinks and tea. Carrying water from home can reduce the need to buy bottled water or other beverages just because you are thirsty.

Enjoy eating out.

Allow yourself the luxury of dining out, but choose the occasions and restaurants, rather than grabbing food because you haven't planned ahead. Think about how eating out fits into your budget and healthful lifestyle. What restaurants in your area offer delicious, nutritious, and affordable meals? Better to eat out half as often but enjoy good food. If portions are large, have leftovers for lunch the next day.

Prepare some meals at home.

If you are short on time, develop a repertoire of meals that are quick and easy, as well as nutritious. Search the web for ideas, or buy a cookbook with simple recipes featuring healthful foods. If you like to cook, you already know how much cheaper food prepared at home can be. When you prepare a meal, save time by making extra for lunch the next day, or portions to freeze.

Shop wisely.

Make a list before you shop, and stick to it. Avoid shopping when hungry or tired. Stock up on sale items (only the ones on your list!), and store or freeze for later. Buy produce in season. Look for farmers markets and other local food producers.

Be sure eating is delicious as well as nutritious.

You deserve to enjoy your food! Eating is meant to be satisfying. If you find you are worrying too much about food, step back and relax. Eat slowly and mindfully, enjoying the flavors, textures, and colors of your food.

The same goes for family dining. If you cook for a family, you will need to balance everyone's preferences, and compromise on many fronts. Don't expect to be perfect, but try to gradually improve the food quality in your home. Be sure meals continue to be relaxing occasions where you enjoy time with family and friends.

Healthful Tips for Eating on the Run

Getting stuck in the fast lane seems to be a way of life for many of us these days. Too much to do in not enough time means little time for preparing and cleaning up after meals, with meal time often leaving us feeling rushed and hassled. Following are a few tips to reduce stress and improve your diet when eating on the run.

Make good nutrition a priority.

Just as you make time for exercise, you can make time for improving your diet. Good nutrition and exercise go hand-in-hand when it comes to preventing and treating chronic disease and improving the way you look and feel. For some people, a few small changes will dramatically improve their diets. Others may need to learn more about nutrition. If you don't know the difference between ice cream and sherbet (the latter is lower in fat), you need to master a few nutrition basics. Talk to a nutrition counselor or ask your instructor for some good reading for beginners.

Eat balanced meals.

Use the food pyramid. Each meal, not just dinner, should contain produce (fruits and/or vegetables), a protein choice (from the dairy, meat or meat-substitute groups) and a grain or grain product. Half of your "plate" for each meal should contain produce, one-fourth protein and one-fourth grain. Make low-fat food choices within these categories as much as possible. Read labels, and learn which foods tend to be lower in fat.

Enjoy delicious food.

Eating should be a pleasure! Delicious food helps us feel satisfied so we don't leave the meal craving more food. Healthful need not mean boring. The most important part of a dish, the flavoring, can be added in many quick and easy ways. Experiment with the hundreds of spices and sauces you can find in your supermarket. Look for barbeque, teriyaki, peanut, ginger, and other ready-made sauces. Use these with meats, pasta, rice, and steamed vegetables. Try hot sauces, ginger, and garlic, all of which are good for your health. Cultivate a repertoire of quick and easy dishes you enjoy.

Make healthful eating convenient.

At home, eating convenience means a well-stocked kitchen, so that the ingredients you need are always on hand. At work this may mean bringing leftovers from last night's dinner to microwave for lunch. People who live alone should keep it simple. If you buy meat, freeze it in single portions. If fresh vegetables end up rotting in your refrigerator, buy in small quantities, and keep extra portions frozen. Cooking for a family? One meal should be adaptable to all food preferences with minor manipulations. Growing teens can eat larger portions; vegetarians can microwave a meat substitute that is always on hand. Make two or three times as much as you'll need, and use leftovers for meals later in the week.

Use the force of habit to reduce stress.

Develop healthful lunch alternatives and make them a habit, whether you take your own food to work or eat out. Ditto for breakfast. For dinner, try a weekly meal plan, such as Sunday, casserole; Monday, pasta; Tuesday, leftover casserole; Wednesday, takeout chicken; Thursday, take-out Chinese; Friday, broiled fish; and so forth, substituting whatever foods you love. The stress of eating often comes from having to decide each day what to eat and having to shop on the way home from work for the ingredients, all the while resenting this "wasted time."

Make your shopping trips as efficient as possible.

Keep a list that corresponds to the layout of your supermarket. Buy key ingredients you always need to have on hand. Purchase ingredients for the meals on your upcoming weekly meal plan. Plan ahead for special events to avoid extra shopping trips at the last minute when you are most likely to feel hassled and rushed.

Make good choices when eating out.

In fast-food establishments, look for grilled chicken (hold the mayo and use honey-mustard sauce or ketchup), subs with no mayo or cheese, baked potatoes and stuffed pitas. In restaurants with more choices, order salads and steamed vegetables, and low-fat entrees. Avoid gravies and high-fat cream sauces, cream-based soups, and fatty cuts of meat.

Eat Your Fruits and Vegetables

Your mother always said it. Now everyone else seems to be saying it, too—from the Department of Agriculture to the American Heart Association: Eat more fruits and vegetables. Fruits and vegetables supply many important vitamins and minerals, as well as dietary fiber. They also provide other important compounds that prevent the cellular damage that is associated with disorders such as artery disease and cancer. These important compounds are found in a wide array of fruits, vegetables, and other plant foods, including legumes (kidney beans, lentils, split peas, soy beans, etc.), grains, nuts, and seeds, but not in supplements. Including a wide variety of fruits, vegetables, and other plant foods in your diet is the only way to achieve adequate intake of these helpful chemicals.

Go for variety in your choices.

Experts recommend two to four servings of fruits and four or more servings of vegetables a day. Some experts recommend nine or ten servings of fruits and vegetables a day, and that you should also try to eat least three different colors of fruits and vegetables a day. Try to eat foods from at least three of these four categories every day:

- Citrus fruits and juices
- Cruciferous vegetables, such as broccoli, Brussels sprouts, cabbage, kale, cauliflower, and turnips
- Red, orange, and yellow fruits and vegetables
- Dark green, leafy vegetables

Count how many servings of each category you eat in a typical day, and rate yourself on the variety of your choices. If you have room for improvement, you are not alone. The following are some suggestions for quick and easy ways you can add more fruits and vegetables, and more variety, to your diet.

Keep a variety of fruit on hand.

Reach for a piece of fruit when you need a snack. Variety increases the value of your fruit choices. If you are stuck on apples and bananas, try something new. What about apricots, peaches, or grapes? Kiwis, oranges, and melons are other nutritious choices. If you live alone and don't want to keep too much fruit on hand, don't worry about too much variety within a day, or even a week. But vary your choices each time you shop.

Take advantage of prepared vegetables in the produce aisle.

Buy vegetables ready to throw into the steamer. Winter squash, delicious mashed or blended into a soup, is easy to use when you don't have to do the cutting and peeling. Too lazy to make a salad? Buy prewashed mixes of greens ready to throw into your bowl. Chopped cabbage and shredded carrots are other time-savers.

Keep frozen vegetables on hand.

Frozen vegetables are often as nutritious as their fresh counterparts. Frozen mixed vegetables make a quick side dish. Add frozen spinach to tomato sauce and serve over pasta. Many frozen vegetable preparations are available for quick stir-fry meals.

Add raw vegetables to snacks and lunch.

Peeled baby carrots and celery sticks can go just about anywhere and make great snacks. Broccoli crowns, cauliflower chunks and sweet pepper slices are other options.

Adorn sandwiches.

Add lettuce, tomato, onions, peppers, shredded carrots, or sprouts to your sandwiches.

Don't overlook juice.

Citrus, tomato and vegetable juices are especially nutritious. But be sure juices are not your primary source of fruits and vegetables. And remember that fruit juices are especially high in sugar and calories, and low in fiber.

Take advantage of salad bar variety.

Most salad bars mean automatic variety. Look for low fat choices, however, rather than vegetable dishes, such as coleslaw, that are prepared with high-fat dressings.

Develop a repertoire of easy-to-prepare vegetable dishes.

Anyone can bake a yam (clean it, prick it, throw it in the oven or microwave) or steam broccoli. Don't let a lack of cooking know-how limit your diet. Many wonderful cookbooks feature simple, easy, and wholesome recipes.

Plan of Action for a Healthful Diet

If you're watching your blood pressure, your cholesterol or your weight, you are no doubt also watching your diet. A nutritious diet is important for maintaining good health and preventing disease. Your goal should be more nutrition per calorie, and probably fewer of those. You may also be avoiding foods high in saturated fats, cholesterol, salt, sugar, and alcohol, and trying to eat more fresh fruits and vegetables, which are high in fiber, vitamins and minerals.

Sounds simple, but dietary changes never happen solely from good intentions. Those intentions must get translated into good food choices and meal planning. Without some organization and planning, those good intentions can get lost in the realities of daily life.

Assess current habits.

Decide what you are already doing well and what habits could use some improvement. Perhaps you have a nutritious breakfast but the day starts to fall apart by noon, so you grab some high-fat fast food for lunch and a pizza for dinner. See if you can detect any predictable patterns. Some people find recording their food intake for three to five days helpful.

A dietician or nutritionist can help you assess your diet and suggest appropriate changes. Once you have a good idea of the meals that need the most help, you can start to plan ahead.

Make a plan for shopping.

Avoid impulse buying, which is often a dieter's downfall. Stick to your list, and just say no to the candy bars at the checkout counter.

Make a list of nutritious foods you want to have on hand for snacking and meals, both at home and at work. Often, we eat foods because we're hungry and we reach for the closest thing. If you make healthful foods convenient, you'll avoid impulse snacking on empty-calorie foods, and make healthful choices a habit.

Read labels.

There is a wonderful variety of convenience foods in the supermarket, but it's important to read labels and buy defensively. Be especially aware of fat, salt, and calories.

Fat content is the hardest to decipher. Avoid foods high in saturated fats. Total intake of saturated fats should be less than 10 to 15 grams per day. Also avoid foods with hydrogenated oils, which can have the same negative health effects as saturated fats.

Beware of "no cholesterol" foods that may be high in fat, and words like "lite," which could be misleading.

Daily sodium intake should be less than 2,000 to 3,000 mg per day. Since salt is frequently added to prepared foods, it's easy to exceed this limit if you are consuming prepared foods. Take-out and fast foods are also usually high in salt.

Make a weekly meal plan.

Plan meals ahead of time, and shop for necessary ingredients. Trying to plan a meal at the end of a busy day can be stressful, and may make you decide that nutritious eating just isn't worth the pain and aggravation.

A low-fat diet must be low-stress as well. Organization is the key. The time you spend planning once a week will save the time and stress of last-minute shopping and help you stick to your good intention.

Planning doesn't mean you'll cook every night. Plan meals around your schedule, which can include late exercise classes or evening meetings. On busy days, plan on healthful take-out food or leftovers. Decide which nights you'll eat out, and adjust the rest of the day's food intake accordingly. A weekly plan can help encourage variety in your diet and give you a sense of control.

Develop a repertoire of simple, quick recipes that you and those you cook for enjoy. Once you get organized, healthful cooking and eating become a way of life.

Evaluating Information on Dietary Supplements

They look like drugs, and if you read the labels, they sound like drugs. When you purchase a bottle of vitamins or an herbal remedy at the drug store or supermarket, you might assume that these products are similar to the over-the-counter drugs in the next aisle. But the regulation of dietary supplements is quite different.

What exactly is a dietary supplement?

A dietary supplement is manufactured from ingredients that could appear in the diet: components of plants and animals. Keep in mind, however, that these ingredients may be concentrated and changed in other ways, so that in the end they bear little resemblance to chemicals that might appear in your breakfast, lunch, or dinner.

Dietary supplements bear a closer resemblance to drugs than food, so you must not assume that just because they are "natural" they are harmless. Even vitamins and minerals can be harmful if you consume too much of them. You can tell whether your product is a dietary supplement or a drug by checking the label. A supplement will have a "Supplement Facts" panel on the label.

Although dietary supplements are not regulated as drugs in the U.S., remember that they may act like drugs, and interact with medications you may be taking. Keep your doctor informed about the supplements you are using.

Can supplements contain doses of vitamins and minerals that are too high?

Most vitamin and mineral supplements contain safe levels, but some consumers may get the same vitamin in different preparations. Let's say, for example, you take a multi, then something for the eyes, something for the immune system, and maybe something to enhance athletic performance. Each may contain zinc and vitamin A, both of which may be toxic at high doses.

If you take several different preparations, read the labels, and add up the dosage you are getting for each vitamin and mineral. You can check the safe upper limits against the charts for Tolerable Upper Intake Levels put out by the National Academy of Science. You can find this chart in a nutrition text or on the web at the Institutes of Medicine website, www.iom.edu.

Keep in mind that many foods contain added nutrients, such as calcium. You may consume orange juice, waffles, cereal, and antacids with calcium added. It is easy to exceed the safe upper limit for calcium (2,500 mg) if you are also taking calcium supplements and consuming calcium in your diet.

I know supplements with ephedrine have been taken off the supplement market. Are there other risky supplements I should be aware of?

While most of the supplements on the market are safe, a few are risky. For example, supplements with kava, comfrey, and chaparral have been associated with liver damage. You can find lists of supplements to avoid at the Food and Drug Administration's website, www.fda.gov/Food/DietarySupplements/Alerts/default.htm.

The advertisements I see in the mail and on the internet are very convincing for many products. If this information is not accurate, how can it be legal?

Many supplement manufacturers are honest and provide helpful products and good information on their use. Unfortunately, others stretch the truth a bit, and some are frauds. The Federal Trade Commission may prosecute companies whose advertising is false or misleading, but it may take the FTC years to get a product off the market. In the meantime, consumers must investigate products for themselves.

Remember that testimonials from users and endorsements by doctors or scientists do not prove that a product is safe or effective. Some people see results simply because they believe they will. This is called the placebo effect. Doctors and scientists promoting products may have mail-order degrees, or believe in the product because they are getting paid a lot of money to promote it.

You can find good product information on several websites. The site www.consumerlab.com tests products to see that they contain the ingredients listed. (Don't laugh; this is a big problem! Many supplements don't.) The commercial site www.iherb.com contains a link to The Natural Pharmacist, which provides detailed reports on hundreds of supplement ingredients. Enter the supplement you are interested in into the search option to get to this link.

Is it safe to give dietary supplements to children?

Aside from a basic multivitamin and mineral supplement, children and teens should avoid using supplements for two reasons. First, there is little information about the long-term safety of these chemicals. Second, most supplements have not been tested in children or adolescents. The effects of supplements may be very different in young people, and the potential for harm rarely is worth the potential health benefits. Similarly, pregnant women and nursing mothers should avoid using most supplements, except for those prescribed by their providers.

HANDOUT 48 — Should You Take a Look at Your Caffeine Habit?

Is caffeine good or bad? There are no easy answers to this question, because the answer depends on many things. Tired drivers would say caffeine is good for keeping them alert. Workers attempting to solve problems in new and creative ways value caffeine's mental boost. People with headaches appreciate the relief caffeine brings. But people tossing and turning in their beds may be cursing that late afternoon cup of coffee. Irritable, stressed out parents may be blaming their jangled nerves on too many caffeinated sodas at the birthday party as they implore their kids to please settle down.

Most adults appear to self-regulate caffeine consumption fairly well. They learn, perhaps through trial and error, what amount of caffeine helps them feel alert and productive, and when to stop before negative caffeine effects develop. Negative effects, such as stomachaches, nausea, nervousness, insomnia, and anxiety, encourage most people to limit caffeine consumption because too much caffeine just does not feel good. Because caffeine is a powerful and habit-forming drug, it's a good idea to periodically examine your caffeine habit. Would you feel better if you reduced or eliminated the amount of caffeine in your life?

Children and teens should limit caffeine.

Children are more sensitive than adults to caffeine's effects. Since children are usually alert enough without caffeine, why add fuel to the fire? If they are not alert, figure out what is causing the fatigue. Both children and teens should limit consumption of empty calorie soft drinks, and replace them with more nutritious beverages, such as low-fat or nonfat milk.

Watch out for added fats and calories in your caffeinated drinks.

Sodas can be loaded with sugar, and coffee and tea drinks can be loaded with fats and calories. Save these beverages for occasional treats.

Reduce caffeine intake if you experience irregular heart beats, anxiety, or insomnia.

Some people experience an irregular heartbeat when they consume caffeine. Their hearts feel like they are beating much too fast, or are "skipping beats." For some people, any caffeine is too much caffeine. Decaffeinated coffee, tea, and cola drinks may be safe for others, since the amount of caffeine in these products is quite minimal.

Many people experience feelings of stress and anxiety when they consume caffeine. This is because caffeine causes a version of the stress response in your body. And to add insult to injury, people are more likely to overindulge in caffeine when stressed, and end up feeling more stressed than ever.

Caffeine is a long-acting drug, so some of the caffeine consumed early in the day is still circulating in your bloodstream at night. If insomnia is a problem, giving up caffeine may be the answer. Some people find that even morning caffeine aggravates sleep problems.

Consume no more than two to five caffeinated beverages a day.

Even if you do not experience negative caffeine effects, health risks begin to appear in people consuming more than two cups of coffee a day, or somewhat larger amounts of tea or cola. (Tea and cola products generally contain less caffeine, so you can drink more before experiencing health problems.)

Switch from coffee to tea if you experience ulcers or heartburn.

Coffee, not caffeine, is the culprit here, increasing stomach acid production, so decaf is no solution. People with digestive complaints should reduce or eliminate coffee. Tea is not as likely to provoke stomach problems.

Women should avoid caffeine when pregnant or nursing an infant.

A high caffeine intake during pregnancy increases risk of miscarriage and low birth weight. Caffeine gets into breast milk, so nursing moms who consume caffeine may end up with irritable, fussy babies who have trouble sleeping.

The jury is still out on heart disease risk.

But it is probably a good idea to limit caffeine anyway, especially coffee. Two substances in unfiltered coffee raise blood cholesterol levels. Coffee may also raise blood pressure, and the level of another marker of heart disease risk, homocysteine, in some people.

People concerned about anemia or bone density should keep an eye on tea and coffee.

The polyphenols in tea and coffee interfere with iron absorption, so if you are taking iron supplements, drink your tea or coffee an hour before meals, and take the iron after the meal. Caffeine increases risk for osteoporosis, especially if calcium consumption is low.

Weight Control

Chapter 5

Jupiterimages

Trying to Lose Weight? Be Sure to Exercise!

You are embarking on a weight-loss program to improve your health, or perhaps to fit into last year's wardrobe. As you think about the lifestyle changes you will make, be sure to incorporate regular physical activity into your day. Studies show that you can lose weight with changes in eating behavior alone, but weight loss is more healthful and is more likely to be permanent when exercise is part of your program. Following are some reasons to make regular physical activity the cornerstone of your weight-loss program.

With exercise, weight loss = fat loss.

You know you want to lose weight. But think for a minute about what kind of weight you want to lose. Most people want to get rid of fat, but keep the muscle tissue that gives them a healthy, toned appearance, and revs up their metabolic rate.

It is easy to forget that not all weight loss is fat loss. Most people equate a change in scale weight with success. Unfortunately, this leads people to value fast weight loss; but fast weight loss is not all fat weight loss. In fact, the faster the weight loss occurs, the more likely it is to be water weight, as water is shed along with muscle carbohydrate stores. Some of the loss also comes from the breakdown of lean tissue, such as muscle and even bone.

Loss of muscle and bone tissue is harmful, especially to mid-life and older adults who are somewhat small to begin with. Muscle and bone mass decline with age in most people, leading eventually to risk of frailty and osteoporosis. This decline is difficult to reverse as the years go by. Loss of lean tissue is also counterproductive to weight control, since metabolic rate is a function of muscle mass. This means that loss of lean tissue leads to a lower metabolic rate and, ironically, more difficulty maintaining a healthy weight.

With exercise, lost weight is more likely to stay off.

You have probably heard that repeated episodes of weight loss and regain can be harmful to your health. When you go through many cycles of weight loss and regain, you are more likely to develop hypertension and heart disease. You are also more likely to lose lean tissue, gain fat around the middle and end up with a lower metabolic rate. So if your goal is good health, you want to be sure that your weight-loss efforts don't go to waste (or to waist!). You want the weight to stay off.

Many studies have shown that regular physical activity is absolutely critical for keeping lost weight off. People who maintain a significant weight loss for at least two years exercise, on average, about one hour a day. They also continue to be careful about their food choices.

Exercise offers many health benefits.

Public health experts urge everyone to exercise regularly, because exercise offers a number of important health benefits. Many of these benefits reduce the health risks associated with obesity and being overweight. For example, while excess body fat increases your risk for high blood pressure, type 2 diabetes and heart disease, regular physical activity helps to improve blood pressure and blood sugar control, and reduce heart disease risk.

Exercise strengthens willpower and reduces stress.

Changing your lifestyle is not easy. Negative emotions and feelings of stress are the most common reasons that people quit following their weight-loss programs. Regular physical activity can help you to stick to your weight-control plan by reducing feelings of stress, giving you energy, improving the quality of your sleep and helping you feel stronger. As your fitness begins to improve, so does your quality of life. Regular physical activity can also reduce feelings of anxiety and depression.

Create opportunities for daily physical activity.

Exercise need not be intense to be beneficial. If your doctor says you can exercise, start slowly and build gradually. Find activities that are convenient and enjoyable, and get a friend to join you. As little as 10 minutes of walking several times a day can lead to significant improvements in fitness and in your quality of life.

50 Lifelong Weight Control: Get in the Habit of Eating Well

The key to lifelong weight control is the development of eating habits that help you eat well and make good choices. These good habits become your defense against what many have called a toxic food environment, an environment that constantly pressures people to overeat.

The best way to evaluate your eating habits is to record everything you eat during a typical day. Note when and where each meal or snack was eaten, and any other relevant information that affected your decision to eat and your choice of food. The tricky part of this exercise is to eat as normally as possible, and to not let the act of recording interfere with your typical eating behavior (I'm not going to eat these chips because I don't want to get out my notebook and write them down…).

Once you have a picture of your daily routine, evaluate what you see. Are your habits helping you eat well? Do you generally avoid empty calorie foods? Do you get enough fresh fruits and vegetables? Are there times during the day when you tend to eat even though you are not hungry? What situations trigger unnecessary snacking? Do you skip meals early in the day, only to be starving later?

Now the fun part. Use your common sense and knowledge of yourself to come up with one or two new habits to replace habits you wish to eliminate. Try to be as realistic as possible, and remember that food should be delicious as well as nutritious. Consider the following as you think about cultivating a more nutritious lifestyle.

Clean up your eating environment…

We all eat in response to environmental cues: the time on the clock, the smell of popcorn, the box of donuts on the table. Think about the places you eat, and how you might reduce unnecessary temptations.

Start with your home. Limit your exposure to junk food as much as possible. If you live alone, keep it out of the house. If other family members insist on foods you prefer not to eat, at least keep these foods out of sight. Put them in the refrigerator or in cupboards or containers. And talk to your family: maybe you will be a good influence!

At mealtime, serve yourself reasonable portions and keep serving dishes off the table. That way you can resist automatic seconds. Remember that leftovers are good to have, and could save you from making or buying lunch tomorrow.

…But not your plate.

Recognize that many restaurants tend to serve very large portions, so you will be happy you are getting your money's worth. But big portions are no bargain if you develop obesity and related health problems such as high blood pressure. Eat a reasonable amount, and take the rest to go. Do you want to supersize that? Just say no.

Eat with awareness.

We often pay little attention to our eating behavior or our food, shoveling a meal down while watching television, reading, or talking with friends. When our attention is elsewhere, we may not notice when we are feeling satisfied, and have had enough to eat. Eating quickly also leads us to eat more than we need, since it can take fifteen to twenty minutes to realize we have had enough.

Whenever possible, take your meals in a peaceful environment. Eat slowly and enjoy your food. Take time to focus on your food, enjoying the appearance, smell, flavors and textures of your meal.

Replace snacking with physical activity.

Instead of snacking when you are tired, take a brisk walk. Run up and down the stairs a few times. Eating because you are bored? Read the paper while you walk on the treadmill or ride the stationary cycle. Work out while you watch TV. Physical activity helps reduce stress while it burns calories. It may also reduce your appetite.

Get used to it.

Opportunities to overeat are everywhere, so limiting your intake is not easy. Cultivating a new habit takes a lot of effort, but once you get used to a new habit, it will slowly become more automatic. It will gradually take less self-control to say "No, thank you," to foods you don't really want, while you enjoy the good foods you choose to eat.

Tips for Lifelong Weight Control

You are probably familiar with the many reasons people find it difficult to lose weight. For one thing, eating is an integral part of daily life. Food, unlike alcohol or drugs, which you can avoid, is necessary for living—you've got to eat. And, throughout the day, you have to make many decisions about when and what to eat. You must learn to cope with a food-filled environment that is high in fat, sugar, and salt.

Losing weight, and keeping the weight off, is difficult because your lifestyle has to change not for a few weeks, months or even years, but for life. Most people can lose weight; keeping the weight off is the challenge. You must develop habits that are comfortable enough to live with—forever.

Losing weight almost always means swimming upstream in a culture that promotes overeating and a sedentary lifestyle. Dieters are continually challenged by situations requiring self-control, and commitments that squeeze out scheduled exercise sessions. It's not hard to understand why most people regain the weight they work so hard to lose.

And, yet, some people do succeed in losing weight and keeping it off. Two secrets of their success are continuous planning and flexibility.

Know thyself: Anticipate problems.

Once you establish new eating and exercise patterns, the force of habit can carry you along. People who lose weight successfully cultivate eating and exercise habits that work for them and fit into their daily routines. Healthful behaviors become automatic.

Problems tend to arise when something interrupts the routine, such as travel, visitors, illness, holidays, parties and so forth. Some people find that certain situations are especially likely to overwhelm their good intentions. Successful losers come to understand what these interruptions and situations are likely to be, and plan for their occurrence. They learn to recognize when a high-risk situation may be developing, and pull out their ready-made plan of defense.

Eventually, these plans themselves become part of the habit. Eating out? You know what dishes to order at which restaurants. Holidays? You know which foods you really want to include and which you can bypass. Bad weather? You know how to move your exercise program to a different location.

Plan to cope effectively with stress.

Negative emotions, such as anger, depression, anxiety and just plain old stress, often interfere with good intentions. When people feel bad, they try to find ways to feel better. People who use overeating to feel better may have difficulty sticking to their eating plans when they feel bad.

Ideally, your healthful eating and exercise habits will help you feel less stressed. Try to include enjoyable exercise activities in your day: take a walk with a friend, work out at a fitness center you enjoy, or try a dance class.

Deal with negative emotions right away, before they become overwhelming. Prevent fatigue-related stress by getting enough sleep, eating well and drinking plenty of water. Take breaks to do fun things, such as watching a funny movie and spending time with family and friends. Staying busy with meaningful and rewarding activities makes you feel good and can also keep you out of the kitchen.

Cultivate a flexible attitude.

Lifelong behavior change requires a great deal of flexibility and adaptation. What do we mean by flexibility? We mean the flexibility to work around the roadblocks that inevitably arise to challenge your plans, and to make good choices within the constraints of daily life. Interruptions to your schedule? Adapt accordingly and adjust food and exercise as best you can.

Most important is a flexible attitude, and the ability to recover from setbacks. Realize that there will be occasions when your behavior is not ideal: You may overeat or be too busy to exercise. It is human nature to view lapses as failures, but remember: they are not failures, just learning experiences. Forgive yourself, and make a plan to get back on track.

Lapses in weight control programs are universal: Everyone has good days and bad days. It might be helpful to use your imagination and anticipate how you will recover from lapses when (not if) they occur. While you don't want to talk yourself into a relapse, understanding that you are human can help you return to your weight control program more successfully.

For Successful Weight Control: Think Lifestyle Modification, Not Diet

We live in an environment that promotes eating too much of the wrong kinds of food, and discourages physical activity. Changing ones eating and exercise habits often feels like swimming upstream, against a very strong current. But it's the only way to go. People who successfully lose weight and keep it off develop habits that help them cope with our obesity-promoting environment.

Lifestyle modification means changing your lifestyle to help you reach important goals. People who want to lose weight, for example, can change their eating habits to reduce their intake of excess calories, and add more physical activity to their days. Lifestyle modification is more likely to lead to successful weight control than dieting. Most people use the word "diet" to mean restricting food intake for a short time in order to lose weight. While you can lose weight on just about any kind of diet, the weight usually comes back on unless you also make long-term changes in the lifestyle that allowed you to become overweight in the first place.

Lifestyle modification is very simple in principle. First, you figure out what lifestyle habits and other behaviors are a problem. Second, you replace the problematic behaviors with new habits that will promote a healthier weight. While this process is not as simple as it sounds, it can be done, and is, in fact, what successful losers do. And even small changes can make a big difference in how you look and feel.

Self-Monitoring: A Lifestyle Reality Check

Lifestyle modification begins with a look at your current lifestyle. If weight control is your goal, keep track of everything you eat for at least three days. You may also wish to record the factors that influenced your decisions to eat and your food choices. Keep track of physical activity, including daily activities such as walking, taking the stairs, and doing house and yard work.

Psychologists call this process of record keeping self-monitoring. Self-monitoring helps you take an objective look at your eating and exercise habits. In some cases, self-monitoring helps people realize they are eating more than they thought, for example nibbling as they cook dinner, or snacking as they watch television. Self-monitoring acts as a kind of a mirror so you get a good look at your behavior.

What's the problem?

Once you have recorded your eating and exercise behaviors for a few days, take some time to review your records. Pretend you are a health-care provider or personal trainer reviewing the records of somebody else. Look for good and bad choices. What is working well? What behaviors are problems? In particular, what factors are causing the weight problem?

People who study behavior change and lifestyle modification look at both the causes and rewards of behavior. You can do the same. Are there certain things that seem to cause, or trigger, problematic eating? If so, can you change the trigger? If not, can you change your response to that trigger?

For example, let's say that several times a week you walk into the donut store to get a cup of coffee, but you end up buying a box of donuts, too. What can you do about this? To change the trigger, could you avoid the donut store? Take coffee from home, or buy it somewhere else? Give up the coffee? Or, could you change your response? Go ahead and buy the coffee, but pass on the donuts? Or buy one donut instead of a whole box?

What have you got to lose?

We hold on to many unproductive behaviors because they reward us. They help us feel good, or reduce feelings of stress. Changing these behaviors may be difficult if you are afraid of losing these rewards.

You may notice in your food and exercise records that some eating is triggered by emotions, such as anxiety or depression. If you are an emotional eater you might try snacking on smaller portions of more healthful foods, along with finding other ways to soothe jangled nerves and celebrate triumphs. If emotional eating is a big problem for you, you might also wish to talk to a therapist who specializes in eating problems.

Physical Activity: Stress Reduction and Healthy Rewards

To lose weight, you need physical activity, at least an hour of exercise minutes accumulated throughout the day. This is lucky, because physical activity not only burns calories, but also reduces feeling of stress, improves mood, and helps you feel more energetic. Try to become aware of the positive emotional health benefits of exercise to reinforce your good intentions. Once you discover that physical activity has many rewards, it will be easier to develop an exercise habit.

Successful Weight Control: Work With Your Body

Most attempts to lose weight end in frustration, disappointment, self-condemnation and even weight gain. This is because people usually try to lose weight in ways that create the very stress and food cravings that ultimately defeat their weight-loss strategies. Successful weight-control programs work with, rather than against, your body. Weight that stays off is a byproduct of a healthy lifestyle that reduces the need to eat because of food cravings or emotional hunger.

Beware of restrictive diets.

Many people find that diets that restrict certain foods and food groups lead to cravings for those forbidden foods. Perhaps it is human nature to want what we can't have. But the craving for forbidden foods may also be caused by changes in brain chemistry. If the brain thinks that food is scarce, it may signal the drive to eat.

Food restriction may also affect the levels and regulation of important brain chemicals called neurotransmitters. Neurotransmitters are chemical messengers that allow nerve cells to communicate with one another. They are involved in all aspects of nerve function, including processes that reach conscious awareness, such as remembering, thinking and feeling.

Serotonin is one of the neurotransmitters that may play a role in food cravings, especially cravings for carbohydrates, such as desserts, breads, pasta and fruit. Many functions involve the release of serotonin, including mood, sleep onset, pain sensitivity and blood pressure regulation. And many anti-depressant medications relieve depression by increasing serotonin levels in the brain. Similarly, carbohydrate intake increases brain serotonin level, which may be why some people eat carbohydrate foods when they feel stressed.

So what happens on restrictive diets? Couple very-low-calorie intake with restricted access to carbohydrates, and you get hunger combined with food cravings. No wonder such diets rarely work!

Work with your body.

Successful, long-term weight loss occurs as a byproduct of a balanced lifestyle. When you live your life in ways that reduce feelings of hunger, food cravings and emotional stress, you are more likely to achieve the biochemical well-being that enhances weight-control efforts.

Enjoy plenty of physical activity. Exercise is the cornerstone of successful weight control for at least two reasons. Physical activity burns calories and revs up your metabolism. But just as important, exercise makes you feel good and reduces feelings of stress and depression that can lead to overeating. People who are successful in their weight-loss efforts almost always attribute their success to regular physical activity.

In addition, physical activity and weight loss help to keep you healthy and help to prevent many chronic diseases. Exercise reduces your risk for high blood pressure, type 2 diabetes, heart disease and some types of cancer.

Avoid fatigue.

A recommendation to avoid fatigue may not sound like weight-loss advice, but it is! People tend to eat more when they are tired, perhaps by trying to get the energy from food that they can't get from their sleep-deprived lifestyles. Fatigue can also lead to stress, which in turn interferes with your intentions to eat well and exercise.

Nurture your "good-mood chemistry" by getting plenty of refreshing sleep, enjoying rejuvenating recreation and drinking plenty of water. These recommendations will also help to keep you healthy and minimize downtime from colds and flus.

What about food?

Include plenty of fruits, vegetables and whole grains in your diet. Look for low-fat choices when possible, but also include a small serving of previously forbidden foods to reduce risks of food cravings.

Keep expectations positive but realistic.

A balanced lifestyle does not mean that you will lose a dramatic amount of weight in a short period of time. Weight loss will be slow, but it will be more likely to stay off.

How to Eat Defensively and Avoid Weight Gain

Most obesity researchers believe that the rising rates of obesity around the world are a result of our changing way of life. Our current daily life requires less physical activity than ever before. Yet, we have not compensated for this decline in daily caloric expenditure by eating less food.

The most important defense against becoming overweight, and the first line of treatment if you are already overweight, is to exercise daily. Daily physical activity confers tremendous health benefits and burns calories that might otherwise go into creating more body fat. It reduces feelings of stress, a leading cause of fatigue and overeating.

In addition to physical activity, most people must resist the daily temptation to overeat. Food is everywhere, and it's easy to eat a little too much from time to time, especially during the holidays, which can result in an accumulation of too much body fat. Following are a few thoughts on enjoying good food while avoiding overindulgence.

Listen to your body.

Your body provides physiological cues that tell you when you are hungry, what kinds of food to eat and when you have had enough to eat. Instead of eating just because "it's there," try to eat only when you are hungry. Try to select the kinds of foods you feel like eating, savor your food and learn to eat slowly so that you can stop eating when you have had enough. When in a social situation where you are required to eat even though you are not hungry, just take a little bit and leave some on your plate. Or better, anticipate the upcoming occasion, and time your meals so that you go without eating for a few hours before the event.

Never say diet.

People who have spent years on restrictive diets often find listening to their bodies difficult, because they have ignored these signals for so long. They may also fear overeating if they allow themselves to feel hunger. Restrictive diets result in strong cravings for food, especially food high in fats and sugars; "forbidden foods" become more tempting than ever!

Our bodies and minds resist food restriction, probably for good reasons. It's impossible to obtain good nutrition on diets that are very low in calories. So, food restriction is more likely to lead to obesity than long-term weight loss.

Keep an eye on portion sizes.

Obesity researchers have proposed that increasing portion sizes are pushing people to overeat. If extra food is on your plate, you may eat more than you should. When eating out, especially at fast food restaurants, don't fall for bargains that promise better value if you order more food. Order reasonable portions of the foods you want, and forget about bargains. When restaurant portions are too large, split a meal with a friend, or take the leftovers home for a meal the next day. If you know you can't resist cleaning your plate, order soup and a salad.

Portion sizes have grown steadily over the past 30 years. An average bagel weighed 2 to 3 ounces and contained 230 calories in the 1970s. Today, the average bagel is twice as large, with about 550 calories. A serving of French fries in the 1970s contained about 30 fries, and 450 calories. Today you get about 50 fries and 790 calories. By the way, a serving of French fries, according to the Food Guide Pyramid, is only 10 fries, at 160 calories. This growth in portion size can be seen in soft drinks, candy bars, hamburgers, muffins and many other food items.

Eat fewer high-fat foods.

Research suggests that our bodies require a certain volume of food to feel satisfied. Fruits and vegetables supply volume and plenty of nutrition and health benefits, with relatively few calories. Hot broth soups are especially filling, but low in fat and calories.

Foods high in fat supply a lot of calories per unit volume. Of course, we need some fat in our diets, but look for healthful sources such as olive oil, nuts and avocados. Stick to occasional small portions of dessert foods.

Keep an eye on beverages. For some reason, our bodies do not appear to "count" these, and we still feel hungry, even though we just drank hundreds of calories. Eliminate calories by replacing some of your beverages, especially soda, with water.

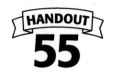

When Stress Triggers Overeating

In addition to keeping us alive, eating serves countless psychological, social, and cultural purposes. We eat to celebrate, punish, comfort, defy, and deny. When people eat in response to emotional drives, such as feeling stressed, bored, or tired, rather than in response to true physical hunger, it is called emotional eating.

Eating and Stress

Stress often throws a wrench into balanced lifestyles, interfering with plans to exercise, eat well and stay organized. Stress commonly affects appetite and food choices. Under stress, some people lose their appetite and forget to eat, while some people remain unaffected and others find themselves eating more than usual, especially more "comfort foods."

Increase self-awareness.

If you tend to overeat when you are stressed, self-monitoring will help change this behavior. Emotional eaters who monitor their eating behaviors often find that the drive to eat masks unpleasant feelings, such as anxiety, depression, loneliness, fatigue, boredom and anger. They learn to differentiate between "mouth hunger" or emotional eating, and "stomach hunger" or true physical hunger. They uncover situations and feelings that trigger overeating.

Address triggers.

If stress triggers overeating, address the sources of stress. Look for solutions to problems at hand, talk them over with a friend, and write in a journal. Acknowledge and address feelings of depression, anger or anxiety. Do whatever you can to reduce feelings of stress.

Most people find that overeating tends to occur in specific places and specific times. A common time is at home during the evening. Possible solutions include engaging in a hobby that keeps your mind and hands busy, such as going out and exercising. If eating occurs, munch on low-calorie snacks.

Exercise daily.

Exercise reduces stress, helps control appetite, gives you energy and improves sleep quality. All of these factors help reduce emotional eating.

Get more R & R.

Fatigue is one of the most common causes of overeating. Getting plenty of rest and relaxation helps manage stress and reduce overeating. Some emotional eaters find that they overeat because eating is the only time they relax, enjoy life and reward themselves. These folks can learn to enlarge their repertoire of "healthy pleasures" so that they have other ways to nurture themselves besides eating.

Avoid restrictive diets.

Diets that are very low in calories (fewer than 1,400 calories per day) or that restrict certain food groups are psychologically self-defeating, often leading to food cravings and too much focus on food and eating. Have you ever noticed that the more you think about not eating the more you want to eat? It's like the game where you say, "Don't think about pink elephants," and of course, pink elephants spring to mind. Such diets also rarely lead to long-term weight control and good health.

Restrictive diets also create disharmony among body, mind and spirit, as eating behaviors become disconnected from the physiological drives that tell you what, when and how much to eat. Overeaters don't know when they are hungry, what foods they feel like eating, how much to eat or when they are full. People must exercise restraint in this environment of plenty. The mind can be a helpful partner, and nutrition knowledge can be harnessed to work with appetites to create a well-balanced and delicious diet.

Make all food soul food.

A heart-healthy diet should nourish body and soul. Food is supposed to be delicious and eating pleasurable. Include your "comfort foods" as appropriate.

Get help.

Emotional eating is so common that some emotional eating is considered well within the range of normal behavior. Problems arise when emotional eating becomes excessive and interferes with lifestyle and good health, or signals painful emotional needs that require attention. If you feel emotional eating is a problem, it may be wise to work with a counselor trained in eating problems.

What Is My Ideal Weight?

Many years ago, nutrition and exercise specialists used the term "ideal weight" to indicate a body weight that would represent both good health and an attractive physique. Researchers derived formulas to calculate your ideal weight based on height, frame size, and body composition. It was thought that people should exercise more and limit their caloric intake in order to achieve "ideal weight," and that having a specific goal weight to strive for would be scientific, helpful, and motivational.

Scientists who study weight control have since learned that ideal weight is not such a helpful term after all, and that weight loss does not usually follow neat and tidy equations. Experts now believe that instead of asking, "What is my ideal weight?" we should ask, "What is a healthful and achievable weight for me?" And some researchers believe we should drop the question altogether and focus on developing a healthful lifestyle that includes good food and plenty of physical activity.

What is a healthful weight?

A healthful body weight is a weight you can maintain with some vigilance, but without severely limiting your food intake. While choosing foods carefully is a requirement for modern life, obsessing about every bite is not. A good diet contributes to good health, so a weight that will not allow you to eat a balanced diet can't be a healthful weight.

A healthful weight may not make you as skinny as fashion models, but this degree of leanness is not realistic for most people. Your weight will reflect your genetic body type. Look at your parents and other close family members. What do their bodies look like? Yours is probably similar.

Has your doctor said that weight loss would improve your health? People who have pre-diabetes or diabetes, high blood pressure, high cholesterol, and other health problems are often encouraged to lose weight. If this is the case for you, remember that even a relatively small weight loss of 5 to 10 percent of your weight can improve these health markers.

Weight maintenance is your goal.

For good health and long-term weight control, maintaining your new weight is the ultimate goal. Almost any one can lose weight with just about any diet. But most people regain the weight within a few months or a few years. Crazy diets, and losing and regaining weight is hard on your body. Ironically, you can end up fatter than before you started to diet!

If you need to lose weight, a better strategy is to lose a relatively small amount, maybe that five to ten percent of your weight, by increasing activity levels and eliminating some extra calories from your diet. Eat well, but get rid of most of the junk, and consume smaller portions. Extra weight will come off very slowly, perhaps only a pound a week. But weight lost slowly is more likely to stay off. Develop a healthful lifestyle that supports your new, healthful weight. Keep that weight off, and celebrate your success!

A better question: What is a healthful lifestyle for me?

Researchers have found that most people embarking on a weight-loss program have extremely unrealistically low goal weights. Many hope to lose 25 percent or more of their body weight. They are disappointed when their bodies resist that degree of weight loss. The resulting disappointment and frustration often lead dieters to overeat in an effort to console themselves. A focus on achieving an unachievable weight can even lead to eating disorders, such as anorexia, bulimia, and binge-eating disorder.

Instead of focusing on a very low goal weight, focus on developing a healthful lifestyle that includes reasonable portions of delicious, nutritious food, and regular physical activity. Successful losers generally engage in some form of physical activity, such as brisk walking, for at least an hour a day. While that may sound like a lot of time, what is more important than your health?

Regular physical activity not only helps you maintain a healthful body weight, it also helps to prevent chronic illness such as diabetes, high blood pressure, and heart disease. Regular physical activity helps you feel great—less irritable, more energetic, and less stressed. Of course, if you are not currently active you will want to talk to your doctor if you have any health concerns, and increase your physical activity slowly and gradually.

The Complete Book of Handouts for Health & Fitness Professionals • Barbara A. Brehm • ©Healthy Learning. All rights reserved • www.healthylearning.com

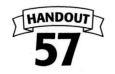

Understanding Obesity Health Risks

Body fat is a good thing, in moderation. But too much body fat interferes with good health in a number of ways. Understanding the impact of obesity on your health helps you understand why it's important to develop a healthful lifestyle: good eating habits and plenty of physical activity. Following are some of the ways that obesity interferes with the maintenance of good health.

Metabolic Interference

Obesity results when people eat more calories than they burn. When you eat extra calories, your body, in its infinite wisdom, wants to store the extra calories for a rainy day, just in case starvation conditions arise. Its favorite way to store extra calories? Fat, of course. It converts extra calories into molecules called triglycerides, and packs the triglyceride into fat cells.

Fat cells can grow larger as more fat is stored, but they cannot expand indefinitely. Weight gain and too much body fat interfere with normal metabolic processes in many ways, ways that contribute to the chronic health problems that are more likely to arise with obesity.

Researchers believe that when people are gaining weight, and their bodies are making extra triglycerides, expanding fat cells may become damaged, or simply reach the end of their life expectancies when they get too full of fat. When this happens, immune cells called macrophages come in to help dispose of damaged and dead fat cells. The job of macrophages is to disarm potential attackers, like bacteria and viruses, by engulfing and digesting them. They try to attack triglycerides and dead fat cells in this manner, but are often overwhelmed by the challenge. They call in more immune cells to help. As more immune cells congregate to deal with the damage, inflammation is the result.

While inflammation is helpful for healing a wound, chronic inflammation can interfere with a number of important biochemical processes in the body. Several of obesity's negative health effects are thought to be the result of inflammation in the fat tissue.

Type 2 Diabetes and Heart Disease

Diabetes may result when some of the chemicals produced by the macrophages interfere with blood sugar regulation. These chemical messengers prevent the body's cells from responding appropriately to the hormone insulin, which signals cells to take up sugar (glucose) from the blood. High blood sugar levels in turn cause more damage, including accelerated aging of the arteries, thus contributing to artery disease, the leading cause of heart disease. High blood sugar also causes damage to the eyes, kidneys, and nerves.

High Blood Pressure

High insulin levels create a stress response in the body, activating the fight or flight response. This can contribute to high blood pressure.

Risky Blood Lipid Levels and Heart Disease

Excess triglyceride production (from excess calories) raises levels of blood fats, including blood triglycerides and low-density lipoprotein cholesterol (LDL) levels. These lipids contribute to the formation of arterial plaque and more inflammation, as macrophages attempt to deal with damaged arteries.

Other Inflammatory Disorders

The inflammation caused by obesity may contribute to other disorders associated with inflammation, such as liver disease, pancreatitis, asthma, and rheumatoid arthritis. Obesity increases risk for Alzheimer's Disease, perhaps through accelerated aging of the arteries. Body fat packed around the internal organs (visceral fat) appears to be most damaging to health. Researchers also believe that inflammation results not only from having a lot of fat, but from getting fatter. Inflammation is more likely to occur when you are in energy storage mode, and your body is dealing with caloric overload.

Cancer Promotion

Obesity is associated with increased risk of many types of cancers. Researchers have suggested that fat tissue may secrete chemicals that make people more susceptible to cancer. Health professionals emphasize, however, that this research is preliminary, and advise that cancer patients not lose weight, as extra weight can be protective once cancer has already developed.

Physical Strain

The physical strain of excess weight can overload weight bearing joints such as the hips, knees, and feet, and accelerate development of the joint degeneration and pain associated with osteoarthritis.

Lifestyle Solutions

Switching your body from energy storage mode to energy utilization mode produces many health benefits. As fat cells stop growing, inflammatory processes slow. A relatively small weight loss (5 to 10 percent of body weight) has enormous health benefits as fat tissue's secretion of disruptive chemicals declines. Consume a heart-healthy diet with plenty of fish, fruits, and vegetables, and increase energy output with regular physical activity.

58 Weight Loss for Athletes: Losing Those Last Five Pounds

Athletes decide to take off a few pounds for many reasons. Some need a leaner physique to enhance their success in sports such as gymnastics, dance, or figure skating where appearance is important. Others hope that dropping some weight will improve their sports performance, giving them more speed or power in events such as running, jumping, or cycling. And some athletes, such as lightweight rowers and wrestlers, have to "make weight" to compete or to gain a competitive advantage.

Good nutrition and a well-designed training program condition your body for peak performance. While achieving ideal body composition may be one of your training goals, it's important to be realistic about how much weight you can really lose. You must also lose weight without sacrificing performance or hurting your health. Following are some important points to consider as you design your weight-loss program.

Lose weight out of season if possible.

Trying to lose weight during your competitive season can have disastrous effects on performance. Better to carry a few extra pounds and have the strength and energy you need to excel. Many athletes find that their efforts to lose those last five pounds leave them energy depleted, unable to train hard or perform well.

What if you are trying to make weight? Experts recommend that you only attempt to drop a few pounds in season, and that weight loss should be fat loss. Dehydration and glycogen depletion do result in weight loss, but are bad for your health and detrimental to athletic performance.

Eat a little less, and exercise a little more.

As you probably know, fat loss occurs when you create an energy deficit in your body, and your body uses fat stores to produce the energy it is not getting from food. Successful weight loss (fat loss) is most likely when you cut extra calories from your diet and increase your exercise volume. Cut out the least nutritious foods (chips, desserts, etc.). Add a little more calorie-burning exercise if you can. But if your exercise volume is already very high, adding more exercise may lead to overtraining. Focus instead on dietary changes and continue your usual level of training.

Be realistic about your weight-loss goals.

Most athletes want to lose fat, not muscle. They may work with a trainer to calculate how much fat they need to lose to reach an ideal body composition. As you think about your weight-loss goals, remember that estimates of body composition are just that: estimates. Even the best measures are only accurate within three to four percentage points. This means if you measure 12 percent fat, you may actually be anywhere from 8 to 16 percent fat. Set a weight range as your goal to accommodate body composition measurement error.

Consume a nutritious diet.

Remember that food is fuel that supplies you with the energy and nutrients you need for physical conditioning and peak performance. Athletes need plenty of carbohydrates to support a high level of energy expenditure. They also need enough protein to make strong muscles and replace amino acids used for energy.

Stay away from diet plans that exclude food groups, especially high-protein, low-carbohydrate diets. These diets do not provide enough energy and you may lose muscle instead of fat tissue. Avoid extreme behaviors such as fasting or severely restricting calories. These cause a drop in metabolic rate, and a loss of muscle tissue, but little fat loss. They also deplete energy levels and hurt athletic performance. Consult a dietician who specializes in sports nutrition (find one at www.scandpg.org) if you need advice on losing weight.

Focus on performance rather than weight.

If your primary goal is to improve sport performance, measure your performance regularly. Keep a record of your race times or whatever measure makes sense for your sport. If you play a team sport, performance in game situations is more important than run times. Ask your coach to help with your performance evaluations.

If performance measures improve, you are succeeding. If performance starts to decline, your weight-loss program may be hurting rather than helping. You may be overtraining, losing muscle tissue, and/or failing to maintain optimal glycogen stores. If weight loss has become more important to you than sport performance, you may be developing a problem with food and weight, or even an eating disorder. Talk to a sports nutritionist or your health-care provider to find someone who can help you regain perspective.

59 Should You Eat Fewer Carbohydrates?

Perhaps you have wondered whether eating fewer grams of carbohydrates might help you lose weight, or make you healthier.

Do carbohydrates make you gain weight?

We get most of our calories from three types of molecules: carbohydrates, proteins and fats. We also derive energy from alcohol if we consume alcoholic beverages. All of these molecules provide the body with energy. Energy (calories) not used immediately by the body is stored for future use. Extra calories mean extra energy storage, and extra body fat. People gain fat when they eat more calories than they burn. Extra calories can come from carbohydrates, proteins, fats, or alcohol.

While fats were the enemy not so long ago, carbohydrates have become the bad guys today. People are trying to lose weight with low-carbohydrate diets, and worrying about their blood sugar and insulin response.

People who have lost weight on low-carb diets often find they begin to gain weight when they reintroduce carbohydrates into their diet. The body stores some carbohydrate as glycogen, a helpful molecule that provides energy for physical activity, and plays a role in keeping blood sugar at a good level. As glycogen stores are replenished after a low-carbohydrate diet (during which they are artificially low), water is also stored along with the carbohydrate.

But sometimes people also gain fat when they begin eating carbohydrates again. This can occur because they have increased their daily caloric intake too much, resulting in excess calories and excess fat. But remember, excess calories can come from any kind of food, not just carbohydrates.

Aren't some carbs worse than others?

Many different types of carbohydrates are found in people's diets. Complex carbohydrates, or starches, are generally healthful when consumed in reasonable portions as part of a balanced diet. These foods include starchy vegetables such as corn, carrots, winter squash and potatoes. Whole grains and grain products also contain starch.

While some foods high in starch do raise blood sugar quickly, when these products are consumed as part of a meal containing proteins, fats and fiber, blood sugar rises more slowly. White potatoes have gotten a bad rap because people worry about their high glycemic index (how quickly the starch from a food enters the blood stream as glucose); but, when a small portion of potato is consumed with other nutritious foods and toppings, it can be part of a healthful diet.

Some carbohydrates are not absorbed by the body and are classified as dietary fiber. Dietary fiber helps keep the digestive system healthy, slows the rise in blood sugar following a meal and helps lower cholesterol levels. Fiber is found in whole grains, fruits, vegetables and legumes (all kinds of beans).

Sugars are found in milk and milk products, fruits, vegetables and in products containing added sugars. While dairy foods and produce contain vitamins, minerals and other helpful molecules, products to which sugars have been added tend to be lower in nutritive value.

Just as people have learned that not all fats are bad, so must we distinguish between "good" carbohydrates that supply good nutrition, and "bad" carbohydrates that have little nutritive value. Diets improve when empty calories and too much starch are replaced by fruits and vegetables.

Are low-carb products helpful for people trying to lose weight?

If low-carbohydrate products help some people reduce calories, then they may help those people lose weight. These products are not always lower in calories, however. They may replace carbohydrate ingredients with fat, and therefore offer no reduction in calories. Some products replace sugars with sugar alcohol and other sugar substitutes that have somewhat fewer calories. In many cases, the products only reduce carbohydrates by a few grams—not enough to make a significant dent in a person's daily carbohydrate and calorie consumption.

The best way to lower your calorie intake is to reduce consumption of empty-calorie foods, such as most baked goods, alcoholic beverages, and high-calorie snack foods such as potato and corn chips. Reasonable portion sizes, balanced meals, and plenty of physical activity are the factors most likely to result in a lifetime of good health and successful weight control.

What Can You Do About Food Cravings?

People experience food cravings as an overwhelming desire to consume a particular kind of food. They crave foods that are associated with positive feelings, foods that taste good, or foods that help them relax and feel good. Researchers doubt that cravings reflect underlying nutritional deficiencies. Rather, the urge to eat may come from a need to improve mood or relieve boredom.

Food cravings are not necessarily a problem, if the craved food is close at hand and you can afford the calories. But cravings can be frustrating for people trying to limit their food intake, and for people prone to emotional eating, since cravings can trigger episodes of overeating.

Prevent food cravings.

Food cravings are most likely to strike later in the day, when you are hungry, tired or stressed. Cravings are less likely to arise when you do everything you can to prevent the physical needs and negative moods that trigger a search for relief.

Avoid fatigue.

When your body needs more energy, you may try to get that energy from food, even though what you really need is more sleep. People who are short on sleep experience more hunger and consume more calories than they really need. And, of course, when you are tired, you are more likely to feel stressed and feel the need to soothe yourself with food.

Exercise.

Try to get some physical activity almost every day. Exercise reduces stress and fatigue, and improves mood. Plus, when you exercise, you burn calories, so you can eat more food—including small portions of the foods you crave.

Drink plenty of water.

You need at least four glasses of water a day, more when you are exercising or in a hot environment. Your body can misinterpret thirst as hunger.

Eat well.

Enjoy delicious food. Select healthful foods you really enjoy. Plan well-balanced meals and snacks that include a colorful variety of fruits, vegetables and whole grains, prepared with the herbs and spices you love. Eat slowly and savor each bite. You are less likely to experience cravings when your diet has a good variety of foods and flavors.

Avoid restrictive diets.

Avoid diets that are too low in calories, or diets that eliminate food groups. These diets may work for a few weeks, but then lead to feelings of deprivation, not to mention hunger. If you need to lose weight, develop eating habits you can live with for the rest of your life.

Avoid hunger.

Hunger can trigger overeating, especially in the late afternoon. Eat regular meals and snacks that include small portions of protein foods, which provide sustained energy.

Reduce food cues that might trigger cravings.

Keep problematic foods out of your home and workplace. Just seeing these foods can set off cravings. Do television commercials make you eat? Watch movies instead. Manage stress throughout the day to prevent the moods and emotional distress that trigger food cravings. Exercise, take breaks, talk to friends and enjoy life.

Avoid tendencies to overeat.

If emotional overeating is a problem, find a qualified professional to help you create better ways to cope with stress or other problems.

Satisfy cravings.

Despite your best efforts to maintain a balanced life, food cravings may still arise. If this happens, take a minute to think about what might be triggering the craving. This information may help you find ways to prevent or deal more effectively with future cravings.

Some people find that if they keep busy, the cravings go away on their own. But others have observed that when they try to not think of something, that something keeps popping back into their minds.

If you can consume a small portion of the craved food without overeating, then go for it—get the craving out of your system. Sometimes you can find a low-calorie version of the food that can satisfy your craving. Perhaps a small piece of dark chocolate candy will do instead of chocolate ice cream. Of course, this only works if you really enjoy the food you choose. Be creative, and look for solutions that are delicious and satisfying.

Can a Personal Trainer Help You Lose Weight?

Scientists continue to study the rising obesity rates around the world, looking for causes and solutions. All agree that changing lifestyles combined with genetic predispositions explain at least some of this increase. People are eating more calories and becoming less active. It takes enormous determination and ingenuity to swim upstream against the currents of our time that encourage overeating and a sedentary life.

Many people who are trying to lose weight turn to a personal trainer to help them stick to their weight control programs. Hiring a personal trainer helps some people make their health and fitness a priority, and improves motivation to develop a healthy lifestyle. The following suggestions can help you get the most from your personal training program.

Check in with your health-care provider.

Let your provider know you are increasing your level of physical activity. Are there any limits on your activity? Be sure to share these with your personal trainer. If you have any doubts, or are unclear about the safety of your program, discuss your concerns with your trainer and your provider.

Start slowly and build gradually.

Your personal trainer will probably ask you to do just a little more than you are already doing, building safely and gradually to a more vigorous program. Be sure not to do too much too soon, and cut back if you have signs of injury. Your personal trainer can help you come up with a program that works best for you.

Figure out why are you overweight.

Do some self-observation and soul searching. Unless you can address the true causes of overweight, your program may not be successful in the long run. If you are overweight because you don't get enough exercise, a personal trainer can help. A personal trainer can also be a cheerleader to encourage you to eliminate empty calorie junk food from your diet, and bring your eating habits in line with public health recommendations (see for example mypyramid.gov).

Is emotional eating a problem? Do you tend to overeat when you feel bad? Is depression, anxiety, boredom, or anger a trigger to overeat? If so, you should address these problems with an experienced therapist.

Ask yourself if you are really ready to change your lifestyle.

Many people feel better when they make resolutions, set lofty goals, and hire a personal trainer. It's almost as though the weight loss has already occurred. But changing your lifestyle is hard work that requires determination and day-to-day dedication. You must be ready to make your health a priority. A personal trainer can give you good guidance and motivation, but you still have to do the work.

Set realistic goals.

Most experts recommend an initial weight-loss goal of no more than 10 to 15 percent of your current body weight. This weight loss should occur in a slow, steady fashion as a result of increased physical activity combined with improved eating habits. Remember that fast weight loss is often not fat loss, but water loss. Fast weight loss is likely to be regained in the near future.

This 10 to 15 percent weight loss, if lost in a healthy way, usually produces significant improvements in health. Such a loss often leads to reductions in resting blood pressure, and to better regulation of blood sugar and blood fat levels. By keeping your goals realistic you can avoid the discouragement that comes when unrealistic goals go unmet. Some people continue to lose weight as they maintain a healthy lifestyle program. Time will tell whether this will be true for you.

Focus on the process, not the product.

Many people find that a focus on the bathroom scale leads to frustration and disappointment, as rates of weight loss are variable and generally slow as time goes by. Measure success in terms of the process (how well you are sticking to your eating and exercise program) rather than the product (how much weight you have lost, or how quickly the weight is coming off). Record your workouts on a calendar, and monitor the eating behaviors you are trying to change. This way you achieve success by reaching your behavior change goals, rather than by weight loss alone.

Use physical activity to reduce feelings of stress and negative emotions.

Lifestyle change can feel stressful. Exercise is the best stress reducer, so use physical activity to improve your mood and energy level. You'll also burn some calories in the process, and enhance your health.

Anticipate positive results, but not perfection.

Sometimes you may overeat, or be unable to attend an exercise session. While you should try hard to stick to your program, life is complicated. Anticipate some disruption, and don't mistake lapse for relapse. Get back on track, your lifelong journey to good health and vitality!

How to Stimulate Your Metabolic Rate

People interested in losing weight, burning excess fat, or both often wonder if there is any way to rev up their metabolic engines to increase their daily calorie expenditure. This information will help you understand how you can burn extra calories and improve your health at the same time.

What is metabolic rate?

Metabolic rate is the energy expenditure required to sustain metabolism. Metabolism refers to the entire collection of biochemical processes that occur in our bodies, many of which require energy. Some of the results of these biochemical processes are observable, for example, breathing and heartbeat.

Most metabolic processes cannot be sensed. Your kidneys are filtering the blood; your cells are pumping substances across the cell membrane and manufacturing proteins; and digestive organs are creating digestive enzymes and processing the chemicals we call food. Following are some ways to increase metabolic activity, and burn more calories each day.

Exercise.

By far, the most significant effect on metabolic rate is achieved with exercise. During moderately vigorous physical activity you elevate your metabolic rate by a factor of ten or more, burning hundreds of extra calories. The more vigorously you exercise, the more calories you burn per minute. If you don't like high-intensity exercise, exercise longer or more often to burn more calories.

Try interval training.

If you like high intensity exercise and are in pretty good shape, try interval training, which allows you to exercise at very high intensities for short periods of time. These high intensity periods are interspersed with bouts of lower intensity work. High intensity exercise requires a longer recovery, which means you burn a few extra calories during the post-exercise period. If you are new to exercise, start slowly and build gradually before attempting interval training.

Do strength training.

Regular resistance training has many beneficial health and fitness effects, such as strengthening muscles, joints, and bones. It can also increase muscle mass somewhat, depending upon your age, sex, and hormonal profile. More muscle mass means you burn a few more calories per hour even when resting. And of course, you burn even more calories during your strength training workouts.

Be active.

Take advantage of opportunities to be active throughout the day. You will burn more calories taking the stairs than you will riding the elevator. Walk your errands when possible. Play with your kids. Limit television viewing, which can actually cause your metabolic rate to drop below your normal resting level (depending upon the show!).

Eat small, regular meals.

Eating small meals or snacks at regularly timed intervals, and eating on a set schedule each day, seems to result in a slightly higher metabolism than eating in an irregular fashion, at least in overweight women. Eating in this way also discourages hunger, so you are less likely to feel deprived, and to overindulge. If you are changing your eating habits to eat more frequently be sure you are not adding calories to your day.

Consume protein with meals.

It takes more calories to digest protein, and a high protein intake may also reduce hunger. Replace high carbohydrate, empty calorie foods with proteins such as eggs, beans, soy products, fish, nonfat dairy products, and lean meats. People with kidney problems should only increase protein intake after checking with their physicians.

Get adequate sleep.

You might think that since you burn more calories awake than asleep, getting less sleep would help you lose weight. Research shows this is not the case. One study found that a shorter sleep duration is associated with higher levels of a hormone (ghrelin) that makes you feel hungry, and greater incidence of obesity.

Avoid very restrictive dieting.

Limiting calorie intake too severely can depress resting metabolic rate. Your body goes into energy conservation mode to cope with a food shortage. This "starvation response" frustrates weight-loss attempts as dieters feel deprived yet lose no weight. While you must decrease your food intake to lose weight, experts usually recommend decreasing your intake by only about 250 calories per day, if your diet is fairly healthy to begin with, and consuming at least 1,200 to 1,600 calories daily.

Enjoy flavorful food and smaller portions.

Delicious food pleases your appetite, so you are satisfied with less. Smaller portion sizes and high fiber foods also help to limit calorie intake. Spicy foods may decrease hunger and slightly increase resting metabolic rate.

Reduce Feelings of Hunger by Working With Your Body

Few pleasures rival the satisfaction of enjoying good food when we are hungry. Since eating is essential for survival, Mother Nature has endowed us with a strong urge to consume tasty food. Hunger is an uncomfortable feeling that drives you to find food. Hunger tells your body that you need calories and nutrients, and motivates you to make finding a good meal your highest priority. Hunger is not meant to be ignored, and trying to work while you are hungry can make you cranky, tired and distracted.

Developing good eating habits is not easy, especially in an environment filled with tempting food that delivers more fat, calories, sugar and salt than we really need. Modern lifestyles further interfere with good eating habits by confusing our hunger signals, and disrupting our sleeping habits and physical activity levels.

People trying to control their weight often set themselves up to fail by trying to control their hunger. They will usually be more successful (and feel better) if they learn to work with their bodies rather than pretending that willpower alone can lead to lifelong weight control. Cultivating good eating habits must be accompanied by an attempt to lead a balanced life. Following are some of the ways lifestyle is related to feelings of hunger, and suggestions for reducing their power over your eating behavior.

Food Choices

You might think that a calorie is a calorie is a calorie, but your body thinks differently. Some foods make your body think it has had a satisfying meal, while others don't seem to connect with hunger level the way they should.

Foods high in fiber, such as fruits, vegetables and whole grains, lead to more stomach fullness than foods high in fat and lower in volume. Warm, brothy soups and big delicious salads help you feel satisfied with fewer calories. It's as though your stomach expects a certain volume of food, and doesn't turn off the hunger signal until this is reached. Many desserts and snack foods are high in calories but low in volume, and are especially likely to lead to overeating.

Meals and snacks that lead to a sharp rise in blood sugar and a fast, high insulin response are typically followed by earlier hunger signals. Meals high in protein, fiber and healthful fats lead to a lower rise in blood sugar and insulin, and delay the return of hunger.

Sleep Habits

Even a single night of missed sleep is accompanied by a rise in ghrelin (a hormone that makes you feel hungry) and a higher intake of calories. Chronic sleep deprivation has become more common over the past several decades, and some researchers wonder if it might be one of the reasons why obesity rates are rising in many countries.

Chronic Feelings of Excess Stress

A lack of relaxation and chronic high levels of stress change your biochemistry along with your appetite. While some people lose their desire to eat when feeling stressed, the majority of people tend to eat more than usual, perhaps turning to food for comfort. Stress not only interferes with hunger and appetite, but may leave people with less time to shop and plan healthful meals, so they grab whatever is near, with less thought for its nutritive value.

Knowledge-Based Work

Several intriguing studies have found that people eat more after performing demanding mental tasks than after sitting quietly. If your job involves challenging mental work (students, take note!), you may find yourself eating more than you should.

Physical Activity Level

Many people are afraid to exercise because they fear exercise will increase hunger. Ironically, people who engage in moderate exercise often eat the same or only a few more calories than they do on days when they don't exercise. People often lose their appetites after a hard workout, and while they compensate later, they still come out ahead, with energy intake more closely matching their energy expenditure. That's one of the reasons why people who exercise regularly tend to be leaner than their sedentary friends.

In addition, regular physical activity can reduce hunger by improving sleep quality and reducing feelings of stress. It improves blood sugar regulation and blood lipid levels, thus reducing chronic disease risk while normalizing hunger and appetite.

After the Diet: Keeping the Weight Off

Success! You've lost some weight. But now you are worried, because in the past, that weight has crept back on. What can you do this time to hold on to your new size? The following are some suggestions.

Understand what caused you to gain weight in the past.

If you have regained lost weight in the past, take some time to think about how this happened. It might also be helpful to think about how you got overweight in the first place. What can you do to prevent these factors from causing weight gain now? Do certain situations trigger overeating? How can you respond in new ways?

Make a plan.

You probably lost weight by sticking to some kind of eating plan, a new way of eating that helped you take in fewer calories than you were burning. How will you eat now that you are done losing weight?

You may be able to modify the weight-loss diet by adding in a few more calories. This is most likely if your diet was fairly well balanced and included all food groups. In this case, the transition from weight loss to weight maintenance is fairly easy.

On the other hand, if you lost weight by following a very restrictive diet, it will be a little trickier to transition to "normal" eating. You may wish to work with a registered dietician or other licensed nutritionist to come up with a good eating plan that provides flexibility while limiting calories.

Be prepared for some challenges.

Eating in new ways can take some adjustment, but you stuck to you diet, so you can stick to your maintenance plan, too. Be prepared for your new eating plan by shopping for the foods you need. Stay busy, and manage stress. Sticking to your plan will get easier with time, as your eating habits become, well, habits, behaviors that occur automatically with little need for self-control.

Exercise daily.

Studies of people who maintain their weight losses consistently find that these folks exercise—a lot, usually 60 to 90 minutes a day. Any activity that burns calories is fine, and your exercise time may be divided up into several shorter sessions. Choose activities that are as convenient and enjoyable as possible. Find an exercise partner to prevent you from procrastinating, or hire a personal trainer. If you are new to exercise or have any health issues, check with your health-care provider before you begin. Start slowly and build gradually to avoid injury.

Squeeze as much activity as you can into your day. Walk your errands, clean your house, and do yard work. Limit sedentary activities, such as watching TV.

Eat breakfast, and avoid hunger.

People who eat breakfast are more successful in maintaining their weight loss. Try to follow a consistent eating plan that includes breakfast and healthful snacks, and prevents the gnawing hunger that can drive you to overeat.

Weigh yourself regularly.

Some people weigh themselves every day. For others, once a week is enough. Expect daily fluctuations of three to five pounds, but if you see your weight creeping up over time, cut your calorie intake a bit. Ending a diet and going into maintenance is tricky, and it may take some experimenting to figure out how much you can eat without gaining weight. In any case, it is better to confront and correct five pounds of unwanted weight gain than ten or twenty!

Record your food intake, exercise activities, and weight.

Writing down what you eat, do, and weigh prevents denial. It forces you to confront reality, and make necessary adjustments. People tend to eat less when they keep a record.

Be aware of portion sizes, especially when eating out. You probably lost weight by eating reasonable portions. Continue this practice! If you are served a large meal, take some of it home for lunch tomorrow, or share with a friend.

Eat mindfully.

Eating mindfully means eating with full awareness, focusing on the smells and flavors of your food. When you eat consciously you are more likely to eat more slowly, enjoy your food, and feel satisfied with reasonable portions. You are less likely to overeat because you are more aware of how much you are consuming.

It is easier to eat mindfully if you eat without distractions. Pleasant company is fine, but turn off the television and put away the newspaper. Enjoy your meals while sitting down at a table, rather than wolfing down fast food in the car, or inhaling a sandwich at your desk.

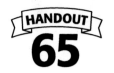

Advice for Healthful Weight Gain

Need to gain weight? Whether you are thin and wanting bigger muscles, have a poor appetite and need to eat more, or are recovering from illness, you can gain weight with a well-planned program of good nutrition and exercise. Your goal is to gain weight healthfully, increasing body mass without gaining too much fat or increasing your risk for cardiovascular disease by raising blood lipid levels.

Step 1: Analyze your current lifestyle.

Before making changes, take a look at your current exercise and eating habits. (You may also wish to meet with your health-care provider if your health is a problem.) Recording your food intake and workouts for three or four days may give you a better picture of your lifestyle strengths and weaknesses.

As you evaluate your lifestyle, consider your stress levels. Stress can interfere with digestive function and reduce appetite in some people. If you think stress may be a problem for you, find ways to reduce feelings of stress. Exercise, talk to friends, watch funny movies, or read a good book. Talk to a professional if stress is interfering with your life.

Step 2: Step up your exercise program.

You want to stimulate weight gain in the form of healthy lean body mass: muscle and bone rather than excess body fat. Resistance training triggers muscle building, so be sure to include a good amount of lifting in your exercise program.

If you are new to strength training, start slowly and build gradually. Consider getting some advice from a personal trainer to get you off on the right foot. If you are experienced, focus on using high levels of resistance. Be sure to warm up before lifting with some cardiovascular exercise, and stretch at the end of your workout.

Some people worry that exercise will make them thinner, but as long as you are careful to increase your calorie intake you should be find. Exercise can reduce feelings of stress and stimulate appetite, and help you eat more as you build muscle.

Step 3: Consume protein and carbohydrate during recovery from exercise.

Strength training stimulates muscle repair and growth. During recovery, your body replenishes muscle glycogen stores and rebuilds muscle fibers to make them bigger and stronger. Consuming some protein (0.5 g per kg body weight) along with some carbohydrate (about 1 g per kg body weight) within half an hour following exercise allows recovery metabolism to work in high gear. "Fast" carbohydrates that get into your blood stream quickly are best, for example fruit juice, sports beverages, sugar, or honey. If you are not hungry after a workout, consider a cool beverage such as a smoothie or shake. Some recovery sports beverages contain protein and carbohydrate.

Step 4: Allow time for full recovery following hard workouts.

Muscle building requires adequate rest and recovery. Alternate hard and easy days, and include one rest day each week. You may wish to perform strength training three days a week, and aerobic exercise on the days you do not strength train. If you strength train almost every day, alternate muscle groups, and include at least one rest day each week.

Step 5: Eat more.

To gain weight, you must eat more calories. Take larger portions and add meals and snacks to your day. Think of snacks as small meals. You may need to plan ahead to be sure good food choices are available when you need to eat. Once you develop a routine, this task will be easier.

If appetite is a problem, be sure to choose calorie-dense foods as much as possible. For example, choose chili or split pea soup rather than broth-based soups. Granola has more calories per bowl than puffy cereal. Beverages are a great way to add calories. Throw some yogurt, a banana, and a little juice in a blender to make a nutritious smoothie.

Be sure to consume some protein with each meal or snack. If you are a vegetarian be sure to include a variety of protein sources to get all of the amino acids (protein building blocks) you need. But avoid too much saturated fat, found in high fat dairy products and fatty meats. Healthful fats—such as those found in plant oils, fish oils, avocadoes, and nuts—are fine.

Do supplements help?

High-protein foods—such as meat, fish, eggs, and dairy products—contain more amino acids at a lower cost than protein supplements. But if you have a poor appetite, meal replacement supplements can be helpful when consumed in addition to (rather than as a replacement for) your meals.

Stress Management and Emotional Health

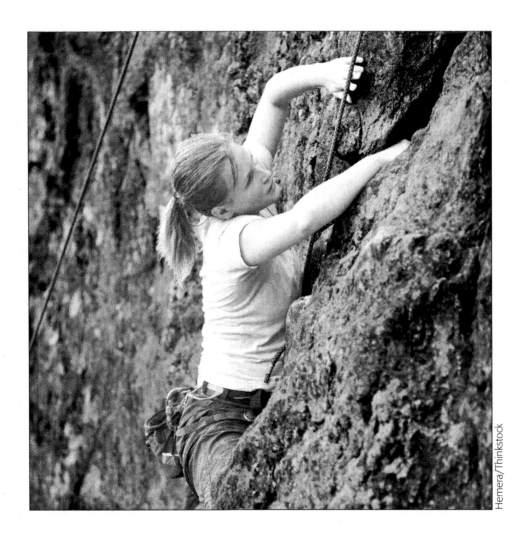

Hemera/Thinkstock

Chapter 6

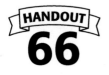

66 Look for Psychological Benefits From Your Exercise Program

Losing weight, preventing obesity, and reducing the risk of disorders like type 2 diabetes, high blood pressure, heart disease and osteoporosis are great reasons to work out regularly. But, did you know that exercise can help to preserve your emotional health, as well?

We take both our physical and mental health for granted until something goes wrong. We overlook symptoms of stress, anxiety and depression until we feel totally overwhelmed or are stuck in a deep depression. As with physical health problems, an ounce of prevention is worth a pound of cure when it comes to depression or stress-related illness.

Psychological Benefits of Exercise

Regular physical activity can help you maintain your emotional well-being, and prevent many stress-related illnesses. Following are some of the benefits of an exercise program.

Reduces Feelings of Anxiety

Anxiety includes feelings of worry, self-doubt and fearful uncertainty about the future. Research suggests that worriers may benefit most from exercise of moderate intensity.

Reduces Feelings of Stress

People experiencing stress may report physical symptoms, such as muscle tension and stomachaches. Others feel emotional upset: feeling overwhelmed, pressured and out of control. Regular physical activity helps to reduce both physical and emotional stress symptoms.

Especially important is that many people report feeling less angry and irritable when they exercise regularly. Feeling angry is the stress factor most often associated with harmful health effects, such as increased risk of hypertension and heart disease.

Reduces Symptoms of Depression

Depression is characterized by a negative mood and feelings of hopelessness. While everyone feels depressed from time to time, depression is diagnosed when symptoms last for a relatively long period of time, or become so severe that they interfere with daily life. Several studies have found that regular exercise of moderate intensity is as effective as other forms of treatment for mild to moderate depression. Exercise is often used in conjunction with medication and talk therapy.

Energizes You and Promotes a Positive Mood

Not only does exercise reduce bad feelings, it gives you good feelings. Many people report positive changes in mood after a workout. These changes include feeling more energized, along with generally positive feelings of well-being.

Improves Sleep Quality

Good sleep quality improves resistance to stress-related illness, and helps you to start the day feeling invigorated and refreshed.

Improves Self-Confidence and Body Image

People experiencing more positive mood and fewer feelings of stress, depression and anxiety tend to feel better about themselves and their lives. Feeling good about what you are accomplishing with your exercise program can help you feel good about yourself. You feel better about your body, as well. Even if it is not perfect, you appreciate all it can do.

Enjoy the Psychological Benefits of Exercise

Enjoying the emotional health benefits of your exercise program can help you become a lifelong exerciser. When you feel too tired to exercise, remind yourself you will feel invigorated and refreshed after your workout. Too stressed to make time to exercise? Remember that exercise will reduce feelings of stress, and help you feel more relaxed, yet alert and focused.

Maximizing the Psychological Benefits

To get the most from your exercise program, choose activities that you enjoy the most, or from which you experience the most stress relief. Highly fit people might enjoy the way they feel after a fairly intense workout. Others may benefit from activities of a more moderate intensity.

Think creatively. Do you enjoy getting outdoors? Exercising with a friend? Or do you need time alone? Would you like to find an activity that offers competition, such as tennis? Or one that requires concentration, such as rock climbing? Look for recreational activities that provide enjoyable opportunities to work out and have fun at the same time.

Tired? Stressed? Think Exercise!

Some people manage to exercise regularly despite hectic schedules, stress and the various demands of work, family and friends. How do they do it? One of the reasons they have an easier time than most sticking to their exercise programs is that they use exercise to help them find balance in their lives, and to reduce feelings of fatigue and stress. Instead of thinking, "I am too tired and stressed to exercise today," they think, "I am so tired and stressed out today, I can't wait to exercise so I will feel better!"

Tired? Stressed?

Many people who feel tired or stressed use these feelings as an excuse to skip their workout. This is understandable. Exercise takes quite a bit of energy and time, and when these are in short supply, it's easy to rationalize skipping a workout.

Psychologists who study health behavior have found that when people are feeling stressed, the need to reduce stress becomes a top priority. The need to feel better now overrides the drive to do something that may lead to future benefits. In other words, if you feel bad and you think skipping your workout will make you feel better, you will probably skip your workout.

The same sort of thinking goes for diets and addictions. If you think eating a big slice of chocolate cake will help relieve the stress you are feeling right now, you are likely to eat it. Stress is the most common reason people resume an addiction they had given up, such as smoking or drinking.

Why not use exercise as a way to reduce stress and fatigue? If you can discover that exercise helps you feel good, this will not only help you stick to your exercise program, but you'll enjoy yourself in the meantime! You will also reap the numerous short- and long-term physical and emotional health benefits that come with regular physical activity. And, if you feel less stressed, you will be better able to stick to your other healthful lifestyle resolutions, such as eating well or quitting smoking.

Discover the exercise/feel good link.

The first step in learning to use exercise to reduce stress is to discover what kinds of exercise make you feel good, and work these types of activities into your exercise program. Researchers have found that people vary greatly in their emotional response to exercise. People who are fairly fit are more likely to find stress relief in somewhat vigorous activities, while people new to exercise may find moderate exercise intensities more beneficial.

In addition to being enjoyable or reducing stress, the physical activities you choose must fit into your schedule and be as convenient as possible. They must also take into account any health concerns you have. (Talk to your health-care provider if this is the case for you.) Your exercise program should also help you work toward your health and fitness goals, such as weight control, muscle strengthening and so forth. If you have questions about designing an exercise program, you may wish to talk to a personal trainer or other fitness professional for some guidance.

Talk yourself into exercise.

Every time you exercise, notice how exercise helps you feel better. If you don't really enjoy the exercise itself (let's admit it, many people don't!), at least notice how you feel better afterward. Many people report feeling less angry, irritable, anxious or depressed. Perhaps you also notice improved muscle strength or more stamina. Maybe you have better balance or muscle tone.

Once you believe that exercise helps you feel better, remind yourself of this fact frequently. When you find you are talking yourself out of exercise, talk yourself into exercise instead.

Strive for balance in your life.

While physical activity is a great stress reducer, exercise alone is not enough. Use the stress-reduction benefits of exercise to help you better address sources of stress. Be sure you are getting enough sleep, eating well, and cultivating the relationships and activities that make life worth living. Seek professional guidance when stress becomes too much of an overload.

68 Taking Stress Seriously

It is almost un-American to take stress seriously. While we have accepted the importance of controlling blood pressure, cholesterol, weight, diet, smoking, and activity level, we are slower to admit that stress could really be a problem.

But stress can be a problem, especially when it settles into our daily lives as chronic, uncontrollable, overwhelming overload. Feelings of anger and depression can be especially damaging. The problems created by too much stress are not "all in your mind." The physical changes that occur in your body when stress becomes chronic are just as real as the changes caused by smoking or a high-fat diet.

How much stress is "too much"?

How much stress is "too much" depends upon your point of view. As Hans Selye, one of the early stress scientists, observed, "We all boil at different degrees." Too much stress for your friend might be an interesting and stimulating life for you, or vice versa.

Stress is not only about what is happening in your life, although that is certainly very important. The impact that stress has on your health is also a function of your perception—what's happening in your mind. For example, you may get anxious or angry about something that may never have happened, but the stress of that anger is very real. So are the muscle tension, digestive problems and chest pain that the anger produces. Or you may perceive a problem in ways that make you more stressed than necessary.

We really can't say how much stress is too much for any given individual. We do know that feelings of anger, hostility and despair can be harmful, so the less of these in your life, the better. Replacing them with humor, optimism and a spiritual outlook will improve your quality of life, and probably your long-term health as well.

Is tension also bad for me?

Some individuals may not feel much anger or depression, but they can still be overloaded and often feel overwhelmed, which can cause tightness while breathing. This sense of tension is bad for your health too.

Chronic stress means your body is in a constant state of arousal from the fight-or-flight response that gears you up to respond to an emergency. This fight-or-flight response is very useful when you need to rescue a child in danger, run to catch a bus or deliver a brilliant presentation. Our problem now is that nature never intended this adaptive response to stay turned on for more than short periods. Once the emergency is over, we need to gradually unwind and recover to an unstressed state.

How can I relax?

What's the best way to get yourself to relax? Balance is the issue. Stress does not appear to be harmful to your health as long as your body has some time each day to recover. Learning to provide a balance will greatly reduce the toll it takes on your health.

The first step in reducing stress is to figure out what is causing stress in your life and do whatever you can to address those issues. A stress-management workshop or seminar might help you learn how to change the way you respond to stress.

Lifestyle is equally important. Get enough sleep, eat well, and eliminate or reduce stress-provoking chemicals such as caffeine, nicotine, and alcohol. Make time for healthy pleasures, such as a hobby, a hot bath or a good movie. Spend time with your friends and write about your stress in a diary.

Daily exercise is the best stress antidote available. Exercise reduces feelings of stress, helps you to relax and counteracts many of the negative health effects of stress. Exercise improves mood and self-confidence, and helps turn those stress mountains back into molehills.

69 Build Resilience With Regular Exercise

A man once worked with his personal trainer to design a good exercise program. He quickly learned how to use all the different machines at the fitness center, and also enjoyed swimming on the days he did not lift. "How often should I exercise?" the man asked his personal trainer early in their work together. The trainer replied, "Try for three times a week, unless you get really busy. In that case, you should try to exercise every day."

Many of us have watched our stress levels rise along with the busy-ness of our lives. Challenging economic times, rising food and fuel prices, political uncertainty in many areas of the world, and job insecurity can leave us feeling anxious and exhausted. The holiday pace can stretch our frayed nerves even further.

When the demands on our time and energy seem to pile up, it is more tempting than ever to postpone self-care, and decide to skip our exercise session today, maybe this week, and in fact, maybe until next year. Yet these are the times when self-care is most urgently needed, to reduce feelings of stress, build emotional resilience, and replenish our good humor and good will.

Researchers have found that participation in regular physical activity is strongly linked to emotional resilience, the ability to cope effectively with the challenges life throws our way, and stay healthy despite stressful circumstances. Emotional resilience is also linked to attitude and outlook, as well as feelings of social support and connection. When the going gets tough, the energy you put into your emotional and physical health pays double dividends, preventing chronic health problems in the future, and helping you cope more effectively with the challenges of the present.

How does exercise increase resilience? In many overlapping ways. The following are a few of the most powerful.

Improvements in Mood

Exercise probably improves mood in several ways. Biochemical changes in the brain and body may help you feel more relaxed and positive. Exercise can also provide a break from work and worry, a time out that leaves you feeling more refreshed and rejuvenated.

Increased Energy

People often report increased energy levels with regular exercise. Even when a workout leaves you feeling physically tired, you may still feel emotionally calm but energized, better able to concentrate and complete important tasks. Most people associate feeling more energetic with feeling better.

More Self-Confidence

Self-confidence may improve when you feel good about making progress toward your self-improvement goals. Some people find they feel better about their body and appearance as they become stronger. Improvements in core strength and posture translate into better, more confident first impressions.

Better Health

You feel better when you feel healthy. You need your health to do all of the things you want to do. Who can afford the time it takes to get sick? Regular exercise helps prevent or control high blood pressure, type 2 diabetes, obesity, and heart disease. Muscle stretching and strengthening are often prescribed for orthopedic problems, such as back and knee pain. Appropriate physical activity reduces aches and pains, and the energy drain associated with disability.

Less Stress, Anxiety, and Depression

Research has shown that regular exercise is as effective as medication for mild to moderate feelings of stress, anxiety, and depression. Everyone knows it is hard to feel good when you are feeling bad. Physical activity can help change the channel on negative thoughts and feelings. Improvements in the body's biochemistry are probably part of the explanation for these positive changes as well.

Improvements in Quality of Life

This is especially common for older adults, who are likely to see benefits in many areas. They may experience improvements in memory and other areas of cognitive function. Strength training may lead to better balance along with stronger muscles.

Development of Other Healthful Habits

Participation in regular exercise indicates a person is making self-care a priority. This resolve to take care of oneself often spills over into other areas as well. People who exercise often develop an interest in nutrition, and start consuming more nourishing foods. They may quit smoking, eat more dark chocolate, or share good jokes with the worker in the next cubicle.

Increased Focus on Fun and Friends

People who make time for regular physical activity often drag their friends and family along. They create opportunities to spend time with people they enjoy, and to have fun.

Meditation: Time Out for Stress Reduction

Once viewed as the domain of cave-dwelling hermits, meditation has shaken off its mysterious trappings and joined the ranks of respected relaxation techniques. Because of its effectiveness, meditation practice is included in many disease-treatment and stress-reduction programs.

Meditation affects both body and mind. By relieving stress, meditation lowers the level of harmful stress hormones that inhibit immune function and interfere with our natural healing processes. And by increasing body-mind relaxation, it eases the pain created by panic and fear.

While there are many varieties of meditation, most include the following elements:

Quiet Environment

Reduce the distraction potential of your meditation environment as much as possible. Choose a time when you will not be interrupted, turn off the telephone and post a sign on the door. If you have a roommate or family, find a time when they will respect your need to practice, and not need to disturb you. A truly silent environment is often impossible. No problem. Background noises are part of real life, and meditation must take place despite real life. Learning to meditate with some background noise is valuable practice.

A Comfortable Position

While lying down is permitted for some relaxation exercises, meditators find the position too suggestive of sleep. A sitting posture produces a more alert mental state. Your sitting position should be as comfortable as possible, and one you can maintain for at least 10 minutes to begin with. Sitting with a straight back, cross-legged on the floor, or sitting in a chair, presents the best musculoskeletal balance, with no one muscle group being made to take all the antigravity stress. During meditation, you may either close your eyes or keep them focused on a point in front of you.

A Mental Focus

Some forms of meditation have you simply focus on your breath. Beginning meditators often use one word or phrase to repeat with each exhalation. Try a suggestive word or phrase like "relax," "peace," or "let go." A short line or phrase from a favorite prayer or poem works well. The word or phrase should help you feel safe, secure and relaxed. Phrases that help you feel connected to a deeper

reality than daily life can help you achieve feelings of transcendence. Transcendence is a grand word for a reachable experience. When you transcend your daily "normal" state of mind, you step outside of the daily grind. You may glimpse a sense of the larger picture, perhaps even a connection to a larger spiritual reality. Whether or not you believe in a god or spiritual power, you at least feel as though you are part of the continuum of history, the web of humanity and life on earth. And if the idea of transcendence is not relevant to your present experience, read on! Relaxation benefits are still yours to enjoy.

Physical Relaxation and Calm Breathing

Meditation practice often begins with a minute or two of physical relaxation and breathing awareness. A quick body scan and a few deep breaths lower physiological arousal and bring your awareness into the present moment.

Passive Attitude

Simply observe with a friendly, nonjudging awareness what is occurring. The harder you try, the more tense you get. When your mind starts to wander, simply bring your attention back to your focus, without judgment, scolding or frustration.

Regular Practice

Like everything, meditation gets easier with practice. Practice is essential for the realization of meditation's benefits. If you are new to meditation, start with one 10-minute session per day, gradually increasing the time to 15 or 20 minutes when you are ready. How will you know when the time is up? Setting an alarm ruins your relaxation. Keep a clock within reach of your peripheral vision, and sneak a glance at it periodically.

Why not give meditation a try? Following is a summary of the instructions previously outlined:

- Pick a focus word or phrase.
- Sit quietly in a comfortable position.
- Close your eyes, or focus them on a point in front of you.
- Relax your muscles.
- Become aware of your breathing, letting the breath come slowly and naturally. Repeat your word or phrase as you exhale.
- Maintain a passive attitude.
- Continue for 10 to 20 minutes.

HANDOUT 71

Lifestyle and Mood: Make Every Day a Good Day

All of us would like to know why it is that some days we simply feel great, and everything seems to go our way. Is it hormones? Blood sugar? Good clean living? No one can say precisely where those good moods come from. Certainly lifestyle is only one small part—but it's a part you have some control over. A healthful lifestyle increases your stress resistance so the bad days are not quite so bad, and opens the door wide so if the good days are knocking, they can walk right in.

Most of us try to exercise regularly and watch what we eat not only to prevent future illness, but to look and feel good today. That immediate payoff feels great and helps reinforce a healthful lifestyle. Are you doing all you can to make every day a good day?

Exercise regularly.

Nothing can turn your mood around more effectively than exercise. Physical activity appears to alter the brain's biochemistry. It makes you feel better and helps combat anxiety and depression. A good workout gets rid of excess tension and leaves you feeling happier and more relaxed. Physical activity provides a diversion from what's bothering you. It helps you sleep better and look better, both of which put you in a better mood. Many scientific studies have shown that regular exercise improves one's ability to tolerate stress and weather the winds of change without succumbing to stress-related illness.

What's regular? Almost daily, so long as you are not experiencing signs of overtraining. Alternate your activities, a practice known as cross training, to get the stress-reduction workout you need, without the musculoskeletal stress you don't. Select activities that you find rewarding.

Check your eating habits.

Food improves mood when your eating habits help you maintain healthy blood sugar level. We've all experienced the fatigue and irritability that can result from being hungry, and the sleepy overstuffed feeling of eating too much. Good eating habits leave you feeling energetic, not hungry and not stuffed.

The influence of eating habits on mood varies tremendously from person to person. You're the best judge of which foods work when for you. A general recommendation is to eat light, high-protein meals and snacks when you need to be alert, and larger portions of starches when you need to relax. Of course, most meals are a mixture of proteins and starches. A lunch for alertness might be a salad with a scoop of tuna, while a dinner for relaxation might be a medium-size helping of pasta, sauce, bread and a healthful dessert. Don't forget to make heart-healthy foods the focus of your diet so you stay healthy, as well as happy.

If you like to feel good and stay healthy, beware of stringent dieting. While keeping a watchful eye on your food intake is beneficial, very-low-calorie diets inevitably lead to food cravings, fatigue, frustration, and an increasing obsession with controlling food intake and appetite. Not to mention a bad mood.

Limit caffeine.

If you drink caffeinated beverages, limit yourself to one or two servings a day, and save them for when you enjoy them the most. Too much caffeine causes anxiety and sleep disturbances. Your body develops a tolerance to a high caffeine level so you end up drinking more and more to get the desired lift. Observe caffeine's effect on your mood and energy level. Heavy users often find that the fifth cup doesn't really give them energy, just the shakes. Play more and manage your stress. When you greet each day rested and refreshed, there is less need for substances that artificially prop you up to help you drag yourself through the day.

Prevent dehydration.

Chronic low-grade dehydration is a common cause of fatigue. And the easiest to fix! Drink at least four to six glasses of water or other beverages (not counting alcohol or caffeinated drinks, which increase water loss) a day, more if you're exercising.

Make time to relax.

You need adequate rest and relaxation to stay healthy and feel good each day. A good night's sleep almost every night is a must. So are activities that allow you to relax and have fun.

72 Depression: Lifestyle Helps Treatment and Prevention

Depression is a complicated disorder with both physical and psychological symptoms. It is a debilitating condition that drains away feelings of pleasure and positive emotions, quality of life, and health. According to the National Institute of Mental Health, about 10 percent of adults in the U.S. suffer from depression each year.

Symptoms of depression vary from person to person. In general, depression is diagnosed when people experience a number of symptoms, including prolonged feelings of sadness or anxiety, hopelessness, guilt, or worthlessness; loss of interest or pleasure in activities once enjoyed; and unexplained changes in sleep, appetite and weight. Depression may be severe or mild, and last for weeks or years.

Depression interferes with every aspect of a person's life. The combination of fatigue, negative mood, and inability to feel pleasure result in a downward spiral of doing less and feeling worse. The best thing for people who are depressed is to get out and do things, but people with depression often have difficulty summoning the desire or energy to do the things that might help them feel better.

Holistic treatment enhances quality of life.

Many treatments help reduce symptoms of depression, and medical care for this disorder has improved greatly over the past few decades. People experiencing symptoms of depression should discuss their symptoms with their health-care providers and make treatment a priority. Because depression has a high rate of recurrence, people should do everything they can to develop a depression-resistant lifestyle, to both treat present and prevent future occurrences of this disorder. The good news: factors that reduce risk of depression also reduce feelings of stress, lower risk of chronic disease, and enhance quality of life, so adopting these measures has many beneficial effects.

But please note: people taking medication for depression should never discontinue it or change dosages without medical supervision. Lifestyle changes complement medication and psychotherapeutic approaches. So if you are experiencing depression, work with your providers to develop a lifelong depression-resistant lifestyle that incorporates the best of medical science and a healthful lifestyle.

Regular physical activity reduces symptoms of depression.

Research suggests that regular physical activity is as effective as medication in reducing symptoms of depression. Most researchers recommend exercise that is somewhat vigorous, such as brisk walking, running, or active sports like basketball or tennis. But studies have also found improvements for people who participated in strength training and yoga.

People who are not currently active should begin slowly, and build gradually to avoid injury, and check with their health care providers to discuss any health concerns. A personal trainer can help recommend an exercise program that will be the most convenient and enjoyable for you. Best of all, find activities that you enjoy and can do with a friend—outdoors when possible.

Natural light may reduce symptoms.

Find ways to increase your exposure to full-spectrum light, at least 30 minutes per day, preferably the same time each day. People who find they become more depressed with shorter days may experience the most relief from regular light exposure. Light boxes can be helpful if you can't spend time in the sun.

Good nutrition supports physical and mental health.

All the good advice you have heard for heart-healthy eating applies to depression prevention as well. Keep your blood sugar and mood on an even keel with regular healthful meals that include plenty of fruits and vegetables. The omega-3 fatty acids found in fish are associated with reduction in depression symptoms. Try to eat fatty fish at least twice a week, and ask your doctor whether fish oil supplements might be helpful.

Get enough sleep.

Try for seven to eight hours a night. If you have sleep problems, follow all the good advice you have ever heard for getting a good night's sleep, such as going to bed and getting up at the same time each day, avoiding stimulants, and developing a relaxing bedtime routine.

Monitor and interrupt negative self-talk.

People with depression tend to dwell on negative thoughts, going over and over problems, memories, and worries, a process known as rumination. With regular practice, you can learn to develop a mindful awareness of your thoughts, and to interrupt unproductive patterns.

Spend time with friends.

It can be difficult to make the effort to get together with friends when you are feeling depressed. Yet this is the best thing for you, for it helps break the cycle of rumination that worsens depression. Develop ways to spend time with people who lift your spirits.

Body Image Resilience

Body image, the way you think and feel about your body, exerts a strong influence on your self-confidence and your quality of life. Many people have a very negative body image, judging their bodies to be below acceptable standards for appearance, and spend enormous amounts of time, energy, and money worrying about how they look. While it is normal to be concerned about your appearance, spending a great deal of your time worrying about your weight and how you look can cause stress, anxiety, and depression, and prevent you from enjoying life. In extreme cases, worrying about one's appearance can lead to harmful behaviors, including eating disorders and drug abuse.

Doesn't some concern about appearance and weight help you develop a healthful lifestyle? Wanting to look good can motivate you to do the right things: eating right, exercising, getting enough sleep, and managing stress. But if you feel really bad about yourself, you may not be able to summon the energy to stick to your healthy lifestyle resolutions. Living well depends upon good self-regard. You will be more successful at changing your habits when you approach lifestyle change from a position of strength.

Why is it that some people make peace with their less than perfect bodies while others become obsessed with achieving an impossible perfection? Researchers have compared these two groups, and have found several behaviors associated with body image resilience, or the ability to feel good about one's appearance despite falling short of society's standards of perfection.

Challenge beauty standards.

This is a nice time in history for naturally slender women to be alive. A hundred years ago they would have been the ones disappointed in their bodies! Fashions come and go, and at this point in time, few of us fit the fashion ideal. No matter how much we exercise and diet, we may never achieve a "perfect" physique. Fashion helps sell products, and encourages us to feel dissatisfied with our appearance so we will buy clothes, makeup, and other products.

Challenge irrational thoughts.

Many people fall for the "myth of transformation," thinking "If I were thinner, I would be happier," or "I would have the perfect mate," or "the perfect job," or "more money." In many cases, people put their lives on hold, waiting until they lose weight to look for a better job or pursue an interesting hobby or travel.

Other people harbor irrational ideas such as: *No one will love me unless I look perfect. I must be a bad person since I can't lose weight.* Replace these irrational beliefs with more realistic and positive thoughts.

Embrace health.

Focus instead on health, and developing a healthful lifestyle to look and feel your best, but not because you must attain perfection. Appreciate all your body can do.

Enjoy physical activity.

Active people tend to have a more positive body image. Exercise for positive reasons – to reduce stress, anxiety, and depression, and to increase energy levels, sleep better and feel stronger. Find activities you enjoy and relish your body's strength, power, health, and vitality.

Make peace with your genes.

Make the most of what you have got. If you need to lose some weight to be healthier, set realistic weight goals, usually no more than a 10-percent weight loss that is achieved in a healthful fashion, and stays off.

Develop your personal style.

The impression you make has a lot to do with posture, confidence, and personal style. Wear clothes you love that are comfortable and make you look and feel good.

Strive for healthy families.

Your family exerts a strong influence on your body image and self-esteem. If you are a parent, help your family develop healthful eating and exercise habits. Model self-acceptance and a positive attitude. Help children get involved in productive activities that build self-confidence. Reduce the focus on appearance. Encourage children to develop "media literacy," an ability to critique the messages commercials send to sell products, and the sociocultural messages embedded in movies, TV, and other media. Help them criticize our culture's overemphasis on material consumption and our under-emphasis on developing meaningful lives.

Cultivate effective coping strategies.

Life is not always easy, but don't blame your problems on appearance. Cultivate effective strategies for coping with stress. Develop friendships that make you feel good about yourself. And get a life! Recognize that health and fitness are means to an end: a life well lived. Get involved in work, recreation, family, and community. Use your talents to make the world a better place.

Helping a Friend With an Eating Disorder

Dieting behavior out of control...obsessions with food and weight...trips to the bathroom after meals...withdrawal from groups and friends they used to enjoy. For some reason, perhaps many reasons, you suspect your friend may have an eating disorder. What is the best way to help?

The best way will depend on your relationship with that person, and the seriousness of the situation. In general, the best way to help begins with understanding. Learn what you can about eating disorders. You probably know by now that eating disorders are not only about food. Eating disorders are addictive behaviors that help people cope with stress and low self-esteem. They are hard to overcome, and can have lifelong negative health consequences.

People with these complex psychological disorders require long-term support from knowledgeable, experienced professionals. The best way to help friends with eating disorders is to encourage them to get help, and to recognize that you can't just "talk some sense into them." But you can let them know you care. You can urge them to face the fact that their eating disorder is harmful to them and those around them, and admit that they need help.

Express your concern.

If you decide to talk to your friend about his or her behavior, find a private time and place to talk where you are both most likely to feel comfortable. Let your friend know this is difficult for you, but that you are worried and feel like you can no longer ignore the situation.

Be specific.

Describe the behaviors that trouble you, and then give your friend time to respond. For example, "I am worried because you've stopped coming to the gym, and I don't see you in the break room anymore." Offer your opinion that the behavior is not helpful, and that you are worried that your friend is depressed or stressed. Offer to go to counseling with your friend, if you are close.

Don't be surprised if your friend pushes your concerns (and you) away.

Unless people with eating disorders are ready to get help, they usually deny or ignore the concerns expressed by friends and family members. They need their disordered behavior to feel okay, and may not see how harmful it is. Like people addicted to drugs or alcohol, people with eating disorders often refuse to admit that there is a problem. Don't let this keep you from expressing your concern; perhaps your words will eventually get through.

Talk to a minor's parents.

If the person you know with an eating disorder is under 18, talk to their parents, even if your friend asks you not to. Tell your friend you have to because you care about their well-being. You can even talk to parents if your friend is over 18, especially if you know the family, but there is less the family can do once the person is legally an adult.

Don't get caught up in your friend's obsession.

You will be most effective if you model healthy attitudes and behaviors. Continue to include your friend in normal social activities. Try to get your friend involved in sports, outdoor adventure activities, community service projects or other rewarding pursuits that might help nurture other interests. If your friend wants to talk, listen sympathetically, without judgment, and without offering quick solutions or providing your own analysis of the problem. People in trouble want emotional support, sympathy and understanding, not intellectual advice. But don't get into conversations about food and weight—that just reinforces the problem. Admit that recovery is hard, but worth the effort.

Don't try to control your friend's behavior.

Trying to control someone won't help, and it may drive you both crazy. People with eating disorders must learn to deal with food. Therapy for eating disorders should include not only some sort of individual or group psychotherapy, but also medical treatment and nutrition counseling. Encourage your friend to get good help in all of these areas.

Take a break from your friend if you find yourself getting too involved.

Eating disorders can be overwhelming. Spend time with other friends, and continue to participate in activities you find fulfilling and enjoyable. You can only help your friend if you stay healthy.

For More Information

Two helpful websites are www.nationaleatingdisorders.org and www.somethingfishy.org. Keep in mind, however, that referring people with eating disorders to a website can do more harm than good, as they may use the sites to "improve" their abilities to control food and weight. Chat rooms on the web can create opportunities to talk with other people who reinforce obsessive thoughts and behaviors.

Exercise and Body Image: An Equal Opportunity Issue

We have heard for years that girls and women may develop a negative body image when they feel their appearance falls short of the ideal. Ladies, move over! Research shows that boys and men also experience dissatisfaction with their bodies. Men tend to wish they were bigger, more muscular but with less fat, while women generally strive to be thinner, but with good muscle definition and "tone."

Increasing rates of negative body image in both sexes appear to be the result of many factors. Climbing obesity rates may be one; as people get heavier, they like their bodies less. Meanwhile, the bodies of models, movie stars, and other media figures have become increasingly unrealistic over the years, creating a wider and wider gap between "ideal" and real bodies. Male models and media figures are often quite muscular and lean, and their female counterparts are quite thin yet shapely.

Some dissatisfaction with one's body shape and size may be normal for both men and women. A little concern can even be helpful, if it motivates you to improve your eating and exercise habits to become healthier. But too much dissatisfaction lowers self-esteem, quality of life, and can lead to harmful behaviors, such as drug abuse and eating disorders, that hurt your health.

How much can you change your body?

Your genetic inheritance and your environment both exert strong influences on your body shape and size. Despite media advertising to the contrary, your body is not infinitely malleable. If your parents are tall and thin, and you are tall and thin, you may never "bulk up" like a body builder. You may increase your muscle size, improve your muscular definition, and decrease body fat, but you may never make the cover of a bodybuilding magazine. Similarly, if you are short and stocky, you can achieve good muscle definition and reduce excess weight, but you may never make the cover of fashion magazines.

Ironically, those who try the hardest to change their bodies, especially to lose weight, often end up the least successful. Too much focus on diet can backfire and cause you to eat more than before. Too much restraint and dietary restriction lead to food cravings and a strong drive to overeat. Too much exercise can lead to injury and an inability to exercise.

It's important to have some perspective and make peace with your body. Accept your genetic predisposition. Exercise for positive reasons: to be healthy, strong, and athletic. Develop a balanced exercise program, and be sure your fitness goals are realistic.

Exercise can improve appearance.

A well-balanced exercise program can certainly improve appearance, especially when you accept the fact that appearance is not just about the physical self. Most people do not have "ideal" bodies, but many are attractive nevertheless. Many factors contribute to visual impressions: your posture, the way you move and carry yourself, your confidence, and even your disposition. Good health and vitality improve your appearance. Regular exercise can help with all of these.

On the other hand, people obsessed with their appearance tend to be less impressive. They are usually more self-absorbed and less interesting. You can probably think of people who are "attractive" by society's standards of appearance, but are not much fun to be with.

Positive emotional health improves appearance.

Regular physical activity can reduce stress, anxiety, and depression. You look better when you are more relaxed! Exercise can help you sleep better, so you feel better during the day. People often report feeling more energetic when they are exercising regularly.

Positive emotional health also helps you "get a life." When we are involved in meaningful activities and rewarding relationships, we become more attractive and more interesting people. After all, a healthful lifestyle is not an end in and of itself, but a means to creating a more satisfying and fulfilling life.

Too Concerned With Appearance?

Experts suggest that some people do become too obsessed with their appearance, and about their diet and exercise programs. How much is too much? You should be concerned if you or someone you know shows the following signs.

- Giving up activities once considered enjoyable in order to eat "properly" or work out
- Developing problems with work or relationships because of devoting too much time to exercise or diet
- Exercising every day, unable to take one day a week off for recovery
- Exercising while sick or injured
- Avoiding social situations because of concerns about appearance, and fear that people are appraising one's body
- Inability to relax and enjoy life because of concerns about appearance

Humor Therapy: The Stress-Reduction Benefits of Humor and Laughter

Most people have an intuitive belief in the health benefits of humor, laughter, and pleasure, but forget to take humor seriously when they find themselves in the middle of a stressful day. Of course, you can't take humor too seriously, but you can probably use it more often to relieve the pressure of the daily grind. Following are some suggestions for maximizing the stress reduction effects of humor and laughter.

Lift your spirits with positive humor.

One of the ways in which humor and laughter exert their beneficial effects is by bringing up positive feelings, such as happiness, affection, and hope. Looking on the bright side of life has many psychological and physical health benefits. If the funny story you are smiling or laughing about puts you in a good (or at least a better) mood and elicits positive feelings, and doesn't alienate the people you are with, then you are experiencing positive humor.

The flip side of this observation is that negative humor is no joking matter. Have you ever tried to discuss something with a flippant, sarcastic person who turned your serious conversation into a joke? This type of "humor" alienates people and blocks constructive problem solving. Also destructive is using humor to insult people. "Humor" can also be used to avoid dealing with difficult situations that really need to be dealt with. On the other hand, positive humor can cultivate the good will and energy necessary to tackle a difficult situation.

Use humor to bring people together.

Laughter brings people together, and sharing a humorous story or situation increases feelings of closeness and friendliness. Some researchers believe that the social support that accompanies laughing with others is one of the factors responsible for the health benefits of humor.

Humor is easiest to use with people you are most familiar with, such as family members and close friends. In fact, your friends may be your friends partly because they have a sense of humor that is similar to yours! You know what kinds of humor these people respond to, so go for it. Has your partner or best friend had a bad day at work? Watch a funny movie. Send funny cards to those you love. Laughter and fun can strengthen your most important relationships.

Take laughing lessons from children.

Children are innately playful, and love to laugh. As we grow older, we laugh less, and find fewer occasions to play. Children will laugh their way through card and board games, backyard sports, and silly stories. If you work with young children, or have children in your life, write down the funny and interesting thing they say. If you have children in your family, be happy that laughing together is not only fun, but it also strengthens your relationship with them.

Enjoy the antics of your pets.

Many people find humor in the funny things their pets do. Almost any kind of pet has its funny moments, and provides pet therapy along with opportunities for laughter. Dogs don't seem to mind being laughed at as long as they know you love them, but your cats might be embarrassed, so reassure your cats that you are laughing with them, not at them.

Cultivate your personal humor resource collection.

Save jokes, comics, cards, photographs, and pictures that strike you as humorous. Keep a list of funny and uplifting movies you have seen, and watch them alone or with friends. You may even wish to buy a few that you don't seem to get tired of.

Enjoy books that are collections from your favorite comic strips; buy some or borrow them frequently from your local library. If your newspaper carries comics, read them daily and save the really funny ones. Send copies to your friends, put them up on bulletin boards at work, and add new ones to your refrigerator collection.

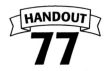

Holistic Health: Body, Mind, and Spirit

Holistic health refers to the notion that people are intricate organisms, composed of a blend of body, mind and spirit. While we talk as though body, mind and spirit are three distinct entities, they are not entirely separate from each other. Proponents of holistic health believe that what happens in one of these areas affects the other areas as well.

In ancient times, healers in many cultures took a holistic approach to health and healing. Prayer, song and worship accompanied lotions and potions designed to heal. In fact, treating the ailing spirit often took center stage as healers tried to help sufferers overcome disease.

Modern medicine evolved in an age of science, and its focus on biological, measurable phenomena has led to many miracles. But as treatment becomes more specialized and high-tech, many people feel like their doctors are missing something by overlooking the "total picture" of body, mind, and spirit.

Although doctors may not do much to treat the mind and spirit while treating a physical illness, many patients seek help for emotional and spiritual needs on their own. Indeed, many people include spiritual practices, such as prayer, in their daily lives. They say that their spiritual beliefs and practices improve their health. And now, after decades of avoiding spirituality and religion as difficult-to-measure and potentially divisive topics, medical research has begun to study the role of spiritual belief in health and healing.

Spirituality can be good for your health.

Several studies examining the link between spiritual practices and health have found intriguing results. A number of practices connected with spiritual health, including prayer, meditation, attendance at religious services and expression of religious beliefs, have been associated with positive health outcomes. These studies have been small and preliminary in nature, but they suggest that, in general, people who have spiritual beliefs and practices heal more quickly from surgery, and cope more effectively with serious illness.

Researchers have speculated on these interesting findings, and have suggested several ways in which spiritual practice might improve health (perhaps in addition to divine intervention, which they have not yet found a way to measure!). Whether you follow a particular religious practice or not, these findings reiterate what many studies have already found from a different perspective.

Social support eases feelings of stress and helps through difficult times.

People need people. We need family and friends to talk to and to call upon for emotional support. The desire to share our hopes and fears is part of human nature. Social support can be found in our families, among our friends, in our communities, at work and in groups to which we belong.

Religious affiliations and other spiritually focused groups can provide a sense of social support and group belonging. In many of these groups, members provide strong emotional support for one another, and in times of stress and illness, people feel comforted by the knowledge that others in the group care. When serious health or other problems arise, members may even provide supportive services for each other, such as meals, housekeeping help, childcare and transportation.

Practices such as praying, singing, meditation, and worship can counteract stress.

Such activities can elicit feelings of relaxation, comfort and wholeness. When we relax, we feel good, safe or happy. Positive emotion leads to many healthful changes in the body and brain.

Thoughts and feelings influence physical health.

Researchers know that some feelings, such as anger, despair, alienation, isolation and helplessness, increase risk of illness. Forgiveness, compassion and love can "open your heart," and protect you from the negative effects of stress.

Holistic Health and Quality of Life

Few people follow spiritual practices to prevent health problems later in life; however, developing habits that keep you healthy in body, mind and spirit can have an impact on your health. Nurturing spiritual wellness, in a tradition that feels meaningful and does not violate the rights of others, can enrich and strengthen an individual's life.

Exercise for Good Sleep: It Beats Counting Sheep!

While those who get it usually take it for granted, people who don't would do almost anything for it. Although it's extremely valuable, you can't buy it. You can't borrow it, steal it, or give it away. And the harder you try to get it, the less likely you are to succeed. What is it? A good night's sleep!

One of the best ways to increase your chance of getting a good night's sleep is to exercise regularly. Many people report an improvement in their sleep quality when they participate in regular physical activity. Studies suggest that older adults and people with sleep problems tend to experience the greatest improvement in sleep quality when beginning an exercise program. (Good sleepers generally do not experience much of an exercise effect, which makes sense because they sleep well already, so there is little room for improvement.)

Research shows that exercise may improve sleep quality in several different ways. Sleep studies suggest that adding exercise to your day may lead to any or all of the following:

- Ability to fall asleep more quickly and easily at night
- Slightly longer periods of deep sleep
- Feeling more satisfied with your sleep
- Less daytime fatigue

Why does exercise improve sleep quality?

Physical activity seems to give your body the message that you need to recover from exercise, and your body responds by blessing you with deep, restorative sleep. Exercise probably helps you sleep better for several reasons. First, regular physical activity helps to strengthen your body's relaxation response, the physical response that is the opposite of the fight-or-flight stress response. Regular exercise relaxes your muscles and slows your resting heart rate.

Second, regular physical activity improves your emotional health. It relieves feelings of stress, anxiety, anger, and depression, all of which can interfere with a good night's sleep. When you feel more relaxed, you sleep better. Exercise may also help improve other physical responses that enhance sleep quality, such as the daily rhythm of hormone and body temperature cycles that encourage deep sleep.

What kind of exercise works best?

The effect of exercise on sleep quality varies considerably from person to person. If you are trying to find out what kind of exercise works best for you, consider keeping a sleep diary, recording your exercise sessions and then rating your sleep quality for that night. Studies show that just about any kind of exercise can improve sleep quality, including cardiovascular exercise and strength training, as well as yoga and other body-mind activities. You may wish to work with a personal trainer who can help you design an exercise program that best meets your Health and Fitness needs, and then modify it as appropriate to enhance your sleep quality.

Does the timing of exercise affect your sleep quality? You may wish to try performing your workout at different times of the day to see if some workout times have greater sleep benefits. Late afternoon works well for many people with sleep problems, perhaps by helping them unwind from a busy day.

Some people worry that evening exercise might lead to wakefulness instead of sleepiness. Evening exercise can be invigorating, but many people find they can still sleep well, even after an evening workout. Others do not sleep well after evening exercise, and prefer an earlier exercise time.

Like most good things in life, exercise works best in moderation. Too much exercise can cause insomnia, so try not to overdo it. If you are new to exercise, start slowly and build gradually to avoid injury and sleeping problems.

Look out for other things that can interfere with a good night's sleep. If you think a medication you are taking might be a problem, work with your provider to adjust your dosage, or switch to a less problematic drug. Eliminate caffeine, or reduce your intake, limiting caffeine to the early part of your day. And, of course, if sleep is a serious problem for you, it may by a symptom of something more serious, so discuss your sleeping problems with your health-care provider.

Exercise and Health Challenges

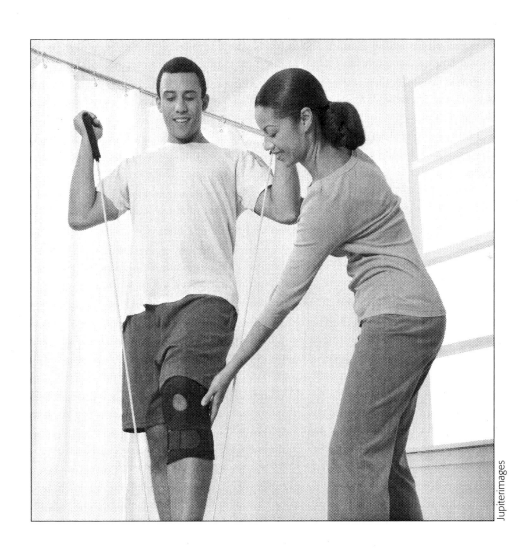

Jupiterimages

Chapter 7

Exercise Is Medicine: Making the Most of Your Exercise Rehabilitation Program

Exercise is great medicine! Your doctor has advised you to exercise to help you recover from injury or to improve your health. Exercise can help make you stronger, reduce pain, and improve your ability to do the things you want to do. Following are some suggestions for making the most of your exercise program.

Be sure you understand your exercise recommendations.

Sometimes exercise recommendations can be complicated. We often think we understand the exercises we are supposed to do as they are being explained by the therapist. But then, when we are trying them on our own at home, we are not always sure what to do.

If this happens to you, remember that this is very common, and don't be embarrassed. Make another appointment with your therapist to clarify the instructions. Be sure all the exercises are written down, with pictures if possible. Take notes to answer the questions you have. You might even have a family member or friend attend the training session with you to help you remember instructions when you are back at home.

Be sure you understand how to exercise safely.

What symptoms indicate that you are doing the exercises wrong, or working too hard? Do certain signals mean that you should skip your exercise program and see the doctor? What should you do if you feel pain? Are some activities safer than others? Can you resume daily activities such as walking and climbing stairs? Discuss these questions with your therapist. Once you know your limits, you can enjoy activity without worrying that you will hurt yourself.

Learn as much as you can about the health problems you're dealing with.

Work with your therapists and other health-care providers to learn as much as you can about the health problems you're dealing with. What can you do to speed recovery, or make the most of your abilities? How can you maximize your quality of life? How can exercise help you?

Report new symptoms or pain to your health-care provider.

If new symptoms worry you, check in with your health-care provider. Pain should also be reported. Many people assume that pain is unavoidable, but pain can limit your mobility and your ability to follow your exercise program. (Obviously, it's also painful!) Your provider may be able to adjust your medications to reduce pain.

Keep your rehab goals in mind.

What kind of improvements are you hoping to make as a result of your exercise program? What will exercise do for you? Set some goals for yourself that you and your therapist believe are realistic. Even small goals give you something to work towards and can motivate you to stick to your exercise program. Some people hope to walk longer distances with less effort. Others hope to regain or maintain the strength to live independently. Many people use exercise to slow the progress of disorders such as osteoporosis, osteoarthritis, or diabetes.

Set up a routine and get with the program.

The sooner you can set up a regular exercise schedule, the better. Regular exercise is safer, and will yield the best results. Exercise will be more rewarding because you will feel stronger faster, and you will not be continually "starting over."

Set up a daily or weekly routine for yourself. If you are supposed to exercise several times a day at home, link your exercise routine to meals, for example, doing your exercises before each meal. Some people do their exercises during a favorite television or radio show, or listen to music.

If you are attending classes or workouts at a fitness or rehab center, be sure to attend as regularly as possible. Work out the most convenient schedule you can, and get involved in the program. The more regularly you attend, the more progress you will make, and the easier the exercise will be. You might even have fun!

Attend regularly and track your progress.

Nothing is more important than your health! Make your health a priority and get the most out of your exercise program. Keep track of your workouts on a calendar, or exercise log. Get a family member or friend to exercise with you. Ask for help with problems that arise. Do everything you can to enjoy your exercise sessions.

HANDOUT 80 — Injured Athletes: Finding Sanctuary in the Fitness Center

Injury is an inevitable part of sport and life. Fortunately, most injuries are fairly mild, and heal with rest and appropriate physical therapy. But some injuries compromise athletic performance for weeks, months, or years to come.

While the physical part of injury is the most visible, athletes know that injuries inflict damage in other ways as well. Injury that limits sport participation can lead to a decline in emotional health and well-being, and compromise quality of life. Most people have a negative psychological response to injury. But athletes have an even stronger negative response than most people, since their lives are so intertwined with their physical abilities.

Researchers have studied athletes' emotional responses to injury. Not surprisingly, athletes usually feel a combination of frustration, anger, boredom, depression, fear, anxiety, confusion, and loneliness after injury. These negative emotions not only feel bad, but also can interfere with your determination to return to play, and to stick to your rehabilitation program. Negative emotions can also compromise your success in school and work, and interfere with personal relationships.

If this sounds like you, it's important to take stock of your situation, and figure out some ways to cope with the difficulties you are facing. Researchers suggest a number of ways athletes can improve emotional health in the context of physical limitations.

Get the best medical care possible.

Good care now means maximizing lifelong physical ability. Get the best medical care possible. Remember that the best care is not necessarily surgical intervention.

Navigating the health-care system can be a challenge, and you may need help making decisions about treatment options. Get second and third opinions from experts you respect. Read about your options in books and articles, and on trustworthy websites. Talk to others who have experience with similar injuries. This work is time-consuming, but may very well pay off in the future.

Stick to your physical therapy program.

Most injuries require extensive physical therapy. Therapy may include visits to providers along with exercises you perform at home. Follow your instructions meticulously and faithfully. Pretend this is part of your preseason conditioning program.

Be sure you understand your physical therapy instructions, including warning signs that you should report to your therapist. What kind of pain is to be expected?

What should you do when serious pain occurs? Most athletes want to know what kind of progress to expect. How will you know if you are getting better?

Cross train to stay in shape and improve mood.

Injured athletes often find sanctuary in the fitness center, where they can cross train using a variety of exercise modes. Even though you may not have access to participation in the sport of your choice, you may still be able to use some of the strength training and cardiovascular conditioning machines. Depending upon the nature of your limitation, you may be able to participate in fitness classes, such as water aerobics, yoga, Pilates, or physical conditioning.

Staying in shape is important to athletes. Your physical condition is a large part of your self-concept. Being side lined by injury is a pretty depressing experience, and watching yourself get out of shape can make this experience even more depressing. In addition, most athletes are used to high volumes of physical activity. Many athletes report feeling stressed and depressed when unable to train. Use the fitness center to continue your training, and you will feel better physically and emotionally.

Remember that your work in the fitness center should complement your physical therapy. Check with your physical therapist to be sure your cross-training plans will not interfere with your rehabilitation.

Expand your involvement in other rewarding activities.

When sport training and competition are no longer a part of your day, your life may feel pretty empty. Do what you can to become involved in other rewarding activities. Whether your role in sport has changed for a few months, or the rest of your life, you must find new ways to feel good about yourself and your life.

Some injured athletes take on new roles for their team, serving as referees, managers, announcers, sports writers, or other assistants. Some volunteer their time at local schools and community centers, coaching youth sport teams. Many athletes become interested in the rehabilitation process, and train for careers as athletic trainers, physical therapists, chiropractors, massage therapists, and other health-care providers who work with injured athletes.

You can also expand your involvement in activities unrelated to sport. Renew your interest in old hobbies you once enjoyed, and join groups with interests similar to yours. Social support improves emotional health, so spend time and strengthen relationships with people you enjoy.

Take Control of Your Blood Pressure

Despite advances in drug treatment, hypertension (high blood pressure) continues to be a major health problem for Americans and people in other industrialized countries. More than half of all people in the U.S. who are over 60 years old have hypertension. This disorder has reached epidemic rates for men and women of all ethnic groups.

Recent research underscores the importance of a healthful lifestyle for both the prevention and treatment of hypertension. Often, changes in diet and exercise habits are enough to control blood pressure without medication, especially for people with mild to moderate blood pressure elevations. Sometimes diet and exercise can even reduce the need for medication, and thereby reduce side effects and lower costs.

If you are already taking medication for hypertension, it's important to discuss your lifestyle changes with your doctor, and continue taking your medication as prescribed. If lifestyle changes result in improved blood pressure, your doctor will want to work closely with you to reduce your dosage in a safe and effective manner. Following are some of the most important things you can do to prevent and control hypertension.

Exercise regularly.

Regular exercise is the cornerstone of hypertension-prevention for three reasons. First, it helps prevent and control hypertension. Formerly sedentary people who begin exercising regularly experience, on average, a drop of six or seven points in both systolic and diastolic blood pressure.

Second, active people have lower death rates than their sedentary friends, even when they have the same blood pressure. Research has shown that exercise reduces risk for cardiovascular and other disease. Exercise also helps prevent obesity, another hypertension risk factor.

Third, regular exercise provides the foundation for successful behavior change programs. Exercise makes you feel good and feel positive about yourself. Stress reduction is one of the greatest benefits of exercise. Stress not only raises blood pressure, but it makes you less inclined to stick to your positive eating plan, your smoking cessation program or your decision to cut down on your alcohol intake.

Reduce sodium intake.

Many people with hypertension find that reducing sodium intake reduces blood pressure as well. Learn which foods are high in sodium, and avoid them as much as possible.

Eat more fruits, vegetables, and grains.

Eating more fruits, vegetables and grains increases your intake of important minerals such as calcium and potassium, not to mention vitamins and fiber. One study found that volunteers consuming a diet (the DASH diet) high in these foods and low in fats reduced systolic blood pressure by four points, and diastolic by three points. This small but significant reduction was accomplished with diet alone, and no weight loss. Add exercise, stress management and weight loss for people who are overweight, and blood pressure reductions often improve more.

Lose a little weight.

Deprivation programs are out! Don't focus on weight loss; focus on a healthy lifestyle. A little weight loss may occur by cutting down on "junk food," eating more fruits, vegetables and grains, and increasing physical activity. Even a relatively small loss, such as 5 to 10 pounds, can reduce blood pressure. The most important goal is the development of healthful habits that stay with you for a lifetime, so that the weight stays off. Weight cycling (repeatedly losing and regaining weight) may raise your blood pressure and be harmful to your health.

Reduce stress.

Reducing stress is another lifelong task. Take a stress-management workshop, develop your sense of humor and read some good books. Develop coping techniques that increase your resistance to stress-related illness. And don't forget the importance of exercise for stress reduction.

Limit alcohol and caffeine intake.

Drink alcohol and caffeine in moderation, if at all. Moderation generally means no more than one drink a day for women, or two drinks a day for men. Caffeine increases feelings of stress for many people, and can also cause a rise in blood pressure.

Control other cardiovascular risk factors.

Since hypertension increases risk for cardiovascular disease, it makes sense to make an extra effort to control other cardiovascular risk factors such as smoking, high cholesterol and diabetes.

Type 2 Diabetes? Think Exercise!

Have you been diagnosed with type 2 diabetes? You are not alone! Type 2 diabetes is one of the most common chronic health problems in the world. Over 1.5 million new cases of type 2 diabetes are diagnosed in the U.S. each year. As obesity rates climb, public health officials predict that type 2 diabetes will become even more prevalent in the near future.

Because symptoms of type 2 diabetes can go unnoticed for years, it is tempting to underestimate the severity of this condition. Eventually, however, high blood sugar levels damage the arteries, nerves, and many organs of the body, such as the eyes and kidneys. Diabetes is the leading cause of blindness, end-stage kidney disease, and nontraumatic (not caused by accidents) amputations in adults. Diabetes significantly increases your risk of heart disease and stroke.

Chronic disease requires chronic treatment.

In its early stages, type 2 diabetes can sometimes be corrected with changes in lifestyle. People with fairly mild elevations in blood sugar are often able to achieve good blood sugar control with lifestyle measures such as regular physical activity and a healthful diet. While these people may eventually go on to develop diabetes in the future, they significantly delay the progression of their disease, and postpone or even prevent the health complications that can develop with diabetes.

Here's the problem: if you go back to your old habits of eating too much and not exercising, the diabetes quickly returns. Diabetes is never "cured," but is rather a condition you must live with forever. Therefore, as you make changes in your eating and exercise habits, think long-term, and develop habits you can live with for years to come.

Check in with your diabetes care team.

If you have been diagnosed with diabetes, you are probably already working with your physician, dietician, and other health-care providers to make changes in your lifestyle that will help to improve your blood sugar control. Be sure to check with your health-care team before making any additional changes, such as adding more exercise to your day. While most people with diabetes are encouraged to get plenty of physical activity, diabetes-related complications may limit the types of activity you should perform.

If you are on medications it is especially important to work with your doctor, as medications must be adjusted to accommodate your exercise sessions. Exercise has potent effects on your blood sugar levels. Sometimes it lowers blood sugar level (by helping blood sugar get into the cells to be used for fuel). Too much insulin and too little food before exercise can result in dangerously low blood sugar. On the other hand, exercise may cause an increase in blood sugar, (confused yet?) since exercise tells the body to put more sugar into the bloodstream to fuel working muscles. You will probably need to test your blood sugar at certain times to be sure your medication is correct.

What kind of exercise is best?

Any kind of exercise that burns calories and is safe for you. Both aerobic and strength training exercise are beneficial. Start slowly, and do a few more minutes each day to gradually increase your exercise time to 30 minutes or more a day.

Try to find activities that are convenient and enjoyable. Many people with diabetes enjoy walking. Others like working out on exercise equipment. Get a friend or family member to join you. The more you enjoy your activities, and the more they fit into your lifestyle, the more likely you are to continue, and to experience the wonderful health benefits that exercise delivers.

The Benefits of Physical Activity

Daily physical activity should be a cornerstone of your diabetes treatment program. Physical activity improves your blood sugar regulation by helping the cells of your body take up sugar from your blood. Physical activity helps to prevent many of the diabetes related complications that can develop over the years. For example, while diabetes increases your risk of heart disease, exercise lowers your risk. Exercise improves your circulation, lowers your resting blood pressure (if it's high), and improves your cholesterol and triglyceride levels.

Excess body fat, especially around the middle, can cause type 2 diabetes. Even a small weight loss can help improve your blood sugar regulation. Regular physical activity along with good eating habits can help you lose some weight.

Best of all, exercise helps keep you strong and healthy, and makes you feel good. It feels great to be doing something to improve your blood sugar regulation. Regular physical activity can reduce feelings of stress and fatigue, and improve your mood. When you feel better, it is easier to follow your dietary and exercise recommendations to achieve maximum blood sugar control.

Heart Disease: Lifestyle Is Key to Prevention

Research on artery disease, or atherosclerosis, the most common form of heart disease, continues to shed new light on this complex disorder. Artery disease is characterized by the deposition of plaque on the artery walls. This plaque, composed of cholesterol, immune cells, calcium and many other substances, grows slowly over the course of a lifetime, and is influenced by many factors. The more we learn about this disease, the more we understand the important role played by lifestyle variables, especially physical activity, diet, weight control and stress response.

A key player in the formation of arterial plaque is LDL (low-density lipoprotein) cholesterol. When LDLs become oxidized, they begin to stick to the cells lining the arteries. The immune system, sensing arterial damage, sends in its white blood cells, called macrophages, to repair the damage, setting off a process called inflammation. Unfortunately, this repair process increases, rather than decreases, plaque buildup. Certain immune cells involved in the inflammatory process increase the likelihood that cholesterol and other substances will adhere to the artery lining. They also cause the cells that line the artery to proliferate, which leads to more plaque buildup.

Not all arterial plaques cause serious harm. The ones that cause a heart attack or stroke appear to do so because they have ruptured. The type of plaque most likely to rupture is called unstable plaque, and has a greater level of active inflammation than stable plaque. When unstable plaque ruptures, blood clots form that may block blood flow, thus causing heart attack, stroke or other vascular disasters.

You can reduce your risk of artery disease by taking steps to slow the buildup of plaque and reduce the level of inflammation in your arteries. Your doctor may prescribe medications for some of these risk factors. In addition, the following are some of the ways that lifestyle can help reduce your risk.

Reduce your LDL levels, and raise your HDL levels.

Total cholesterol level does not tell the whole story about risk of artery disease. Also important are the kinds of cholesterol found in the blood stream. The higher your LDL level, the greater your risk, because there are more LDLs ready to contribute to plaque buildup. Optimal LDL levels are under 100 mg/dL, and under 130 is considered close to optimal. HDL (high-density lipoprotein) cholesterol reduces artery disease risk. HDLs under 40 are considered risky.

A heart-healthy diet can help lower LDL levels. Consume plenty of fruits, vegetables and whole grains, and replace saturated, trans and polyunsaturated fats with monounsaturated and omega-3 fatty acids. How do you do this? Reduce your intake of animal fat and high-fat dairy products, along with processed foods that contain hydrogenated oils (read the label). Use olive oil and canola oil when cooking, and increase your consumption of fish.

Regular physical activity is the best way to raise HDL levels. A heart-healthy diet combined with physical activity may help you lose a little weight (if overweight), which can also improve LDL levels.

Reduce LDL damage.

Some lifestyle behaviors, especially smoking, increase LDL damage by causing oxidation reactions. These reactions activate LDL to form plaque. To reduce LDL damage, don't smoke, and avoid secondhand smoke. Many fruits and vegetables provide helpful chemicals called antioxidants that may help prevent LDL damage.

Reduce artery inflammation.

Smoking and weight gain have been associated with an increased level of inflammation, while regular physical activity and a heart-healthy diet with plenty of omega-3 fatty acids seem to reduce inflammation. (Note: even if quitting smoking leads to some weight gain, you are still much better off in terms of heart disease risk!)

Reduce artery damage.

Several factors increase artery disease risk by accelerating arterial damage. Smoking introduces many harmful chemicals into the blood stream. Another risk factor is high blood pressure. Researchers now believe that even high-normal levels increase risk somewhat. The same goes for blood sugar levels; even somewhat elevated levels speed up arterial damage.

Fight Arthritis With Physical Activity

Joints need movement to stay as healthy as possible. Even joints damaged by arthritis need movement. Activity helps to strengthen joints and keep them lubricated. Moderate physical activity has even been shown to reduce pain for most people who have either rheumatoid or osteoarthritis.

Staying physically active with arthritis is a balancing act, however. You want to provide a healthy challenge for your joints and muscles so they get stronger and healthier. But at the same time you must start slowly and build gradually so that you do not cause increased pain or injury.

How do we know physical activity is safe and beneficial?

Dozens of scientific studies have evaluated the effect of different types of physical activity on joint function and pain levels of people with arthritis. Study after study confirms the beneficial effects of regular physical activity.

We know that without activity, even healthy joints become weaker. With activity, joint structures become stronger. Many people think muscles when they think strength, and of course muscles do get stronger when they are exercised. But did you know that ligaments, tendons, joint capsules, and bones get stronger, too? Activity can even strengthen cartilage, the tissue that covers the ends of bones in a joint. Exercise stimulates the production of the joint's fluid (synovial fluid) that nourishes cartilage. Since cartilage does not have a blood supply, this fluid is essential for its health and repair.

How does activity reduce pain?

Many people with arthritis try to limit their pain medication to avoid risk of side effects. Becoming more active has helped many people with arthritis to reduce their medication dosages. Of course you will want to work with your doctor to be sure you are getting the best medicine possible to help you safely reduce arthritis pain.

Researchers think that activity may reduce feelings of pain in a number of ways. First of all, stronger joints are healthier. Stronger, healthier joints mean you can do more with less pain. While the arthritis is still there, the joint is working better. Physical activity may even help to delay the progression of arthritis.

When people become more active, they often feel better psychologically. People who feel better feel less pain. Some people with arthritis feel they can do more and

that they have more energy once they become more active. This in itself may help them cope better with arthritis pain.

Physical activity has beneficial "side effects."

While physical activity is helping to keep your joints as healthy as possible, it can also help to prevent the aches and pains caused by muscle weakness, such as neck and back pain. Physical activity can also help to prevent weight gain, high cholesterol, and high blood pressure. Activity can help strengthen your bones and keep your heart working well.

As you get stronger, your balance improves. Better strength and balance mean you are less likely to fall. If you are doing a variety of activities as part of your therapy, you may even find that your coordination improves as well. Best of all, physical activity improves mood.

What kinds of activities are best?

The best way to find out which kinds of activities would be most helpful for you is to work with your physical therapist. Your doctor should be able to help you find a good therapist who is knowledgeable about arthritis. Your goal is to figure out what you can do, and then do a little more each week.

Some people with arthritis have limited mobility. But even people who cannot walk can do helpful stretching and strengthening exercises in a chair or in a pool. Many people with arthritis enjoy a variety of activities.

Activities in which muscles must exert force against a resistance increase joint strength, and help people with arthritis. Resistance can be supplied by many things, including weights, body weight, elastic bands, and water. Regular activities that increase muscle strength help people with arthritis accomplish tasks they once found difficult, such as getting out of a chair, lifting objects, or climbing stairs.

Similarly, doing a little bit more walking every day can increase stamina and endurance. So many daily activities require walking that any improvement in endurance allows people to do more things.

Some fitness and recreation centers offer activity programs for older adults that help increase core strength and functional balance. They may use special equipment such as large balls to challenge muscles in new ways. These programs can also be a nice change from exercising at home.

Exercising Safely With Fibromyalgia

When your muscles ache, and your whole body feels overwhelmed with fatigue, probably the last thing on your mind is getting to the gym for a good workout. Usually pain and fatigue indicate that rest is best, as when you are coming down with the flu, or have been injured. It's a healthy signal that tells your body the right thing to do.

This is not the case, however, with chronic illnesses such as arthritis, chronic fatigue syndrome and fibromyalgia. Ironically, too much rest and too little activity can actually make these conditions worse. Without physical activity, the phrase "use it, or lose it" takes on meaning. Bones, muscles and joints become weaker, and flexibility declines. The more you rest, the weaker your body becomes.

Exercise Benefits

Appropriate levels of physical activity for people with fibromyalgia can do more than help prevent further loss of functional capacity. Studies have found that after several weeks of physical activity, exercisers with fibromyalgia report a reduction in pain level, even in tender-point areas. Some of this pain reduction may be attributable to sleep improvements. Better sleep is probably also responsible for the lower levels of fatigue and improved moods reported by exercisers when compared to control groups.

Regular physical activity is a potent stress reducer, and its stress-reduction properties seem to work just as well for people with chronic illness as they do for people who are apparently healthy. Researchers comparing people with fibromyalgia who exercise to those who don't have found a significant reduction in depression and improved general health in exercising subjects.

Exercise confers numerous long-term health benefits, such as better blood sugar and blood pressure control. It reduces risk of heart disease, obesity and certain types of cancer. Some people with fibromyalgia have found that regular physical activity helps reduce the frequency and severity of ancillary symptoms such as irritable bowel disorders and tension headaches.

What exercises are best?

The best type of exercise for people with fibromyalgia varies from person to person. No one medication or therapy is effective for all fibromyalgia patients, and most patients go through months and even years of trial and error experimentation to discover which treatments are most effective for their particular needs.

To find what is best for you, consult with your health-care provider. Their recommendations should take into account the limitations imposed by your pain level, as well as any other health concerns you might have. Assuming your doctor has given you the green light to begin exercising, the best approach is to start by doing a little bit more activity than you usually do. For example, if you currently walk for 20 minutes throughout the day, add a 10-minute walk. Start slowly and progress gradually. Your goal is to exercise in ways that do not leave your muscles sore and tired, so slow and steady wins the race.

Over time, consider including three types of exercise in your weekly routine: aerobic exercise, strength training, and stretching. Aerobic exercise includes activities that involve continuous movement, such as walking, water exercise, and stationary cycling. Select activities that are most convenient and appealing to you.

Strength training includes exercises that increase muscle and joint strength, such as weight training and calisthenics. If you are new to strength training, consider joining a class for older adults, or working with a personal trainer who can help you design a simple, low-intensity program that will not aggravate muscle pain or fatigue. Just a few simple exercises performed two or three times a week can help reduce fibromyalgia symptoms, according to recent research.

Stretching exercises can be performed for 10 to 15 minutes after aerobic or strength-training activities. Stretching helps to preserve flexibility and may help relax your muscles.

Keep an exercise log to help you figure out which types of exercise work best for you, and keep in touch with your health-care providers. Cut back if exercise increases pain or fatigue. To stay motivated and increase the fun factor, find a friend who will exercise with you. Patience and perseverance will help you gain control as you face the difficult and rewarding challenge of adding more activity to your life.

Physical Activity for People With Chronic Pain

Chronic pain enters people's lives in many ways. Sometimes it follows injury. Other times it accompanies chronic illness such as arthritis or fibromyalgia. Sometimes it has no good explanation at all.

Pain is normally a signal to take it easy and allow injuries to heal and illnesses to pass. But what happens when the pain does not go away? Pain specialists can provide medications, therapies, and guidelines for coping with pain. One of their recommendations is usually to get moving.

Long periods of rest or low activity are harmful to the body. Disuse allows muscles and joints to atrophy. Endurance, strength, and flexibility decline, along with quality of life as people in pain are able to do less and less, and their lives can become dominated by disability. Ironically, too much rest increases pain.

Activity, on the other hand, improves circulation and the health of the muscles, joints, and bones. Joints love compression, and the way activity moves the joint fluid around to help lubricate painful joints. Muscles love to contract and stretch. The heart, lungs, and blood respond to an exercise challenge by becoming healthier as well.

If you live with chronic pain, and are trying to increase your level of physical activity, it is important to start slowly and build gradually so that activity helps you feel better, not worse. Adding activity is often difficult, but worth the effort as you take charge of your life and make the most of your abilities, participating in the activities that give life meaning for you.

Follow your health-care providers' recommendations.

The first step in becoming more active is to understand what is causing pain, and what types of activities are recommended. Each person is unique, so you must become the expert on your pain. The providers you are working with, including your physical and/or occupational therapists can help you understand what kinds of movements should be avoided, and which are good for you. Your providers may also recommend the use of ice, medication, and other treatments in conjunction with physical activity.

In order to increase your activity level, you must be confident that activity is not causing harm. When you fear you are in danger, pain increases. When you know that the movements are good for you, you may be able to tolerate some pain, knowing that the activity is helpful, not harmful.

If new pain occurs at any time, be sure to check in with your provider to figure out the cause.

Learn about pain.

Pain is very complicated, and involves not only injured or stressed tissues but also many parts of the brain. Your perception of pain is influenced by many factors, including your expectations, emotions, beliefs, friends, family, and attitudes. Your brain may subconsciously develop new nerve networks that make you more aware of pain. On the other hand, your brain can also develop connections that lessen your perception of pain.

This is not to say you can think your pain away. But many people find that they can reduce the control pain has on their lives by increasing their involvement in activities they like and trying to enjoy life as much as possible. A good laugh, for example, has greater pain killing ability than any medication.

Increasing activity level: Start slowly.

Once you have gotten good advice on which activities might work best for you, decide which to pursue. What can most help increase your enjoyment of life? Which are most convenient, appealing, or beneficial? Do you enjoy water exercise, and have access to a pool? Can you use weights or stretchy bands at home? Or would you like to walk outdoors, perhaps with walking poles?

Begin by figuring out how much you can do without making your pain worse, either during or after the activity. Don't worry if this is a very small amount. This is the amount you should do at first. On the next day, increase the amount slightly. For example, if you can walk for five minutes with no increase in pain or pain flare-ups, the next day walk for five and half minutes. Do this for a few days, and then increase to six minutes.

Keep a record of your activity, and be patient. Avoid overdoing it, or pain may keep you away from activity for several days, reversing your good progress. Slowly but surely wins this race.

Recommended Reading:

Butler, David S., and G. Lorimer Moseley. Explain Pain. Adelaide, Australia: Noigroup Publications, 2003.

87 Coming Back After a Heart Attack or Heart Surgery: The Importance of Cardiac Rehabilitation

People leaving the hospital after treatment for a heart attack, or after heart surgery, are usually relieved to be alive, and to think that the worst part is over. But when they leave the hospital, they are just beginning the recovery process, a process which may take many months, and which may be the beginning of a new lifestyle. If you have been through a heart disease diagnosis, or if you have helped a close friend or family member cope with such a diagnosis, you know what a challenge this can be.

Cardiac rehabilitation refers to the activities and lifestyle changes that people are told to make or decide to make following a heart attack or heart surgery. The purpose of cardiac rehabilitation programs are to help people return to everyday life, and hopefully to prevent a heart attack (or another heart attack) and halt or slow disease progression. Cardiac rehabilitation helps people achieve their highest potential for physical and psychological well-being.

I thought cardiac rehabilitation programs were mainly exercise programs.

Exercise is the cornerstone for most exercise rehabilitation programs. People recovering from heart disease are often afraid that physical exertion will be too stressful for their hearts. To recover from heart disease, people must be able to participate in appropriate levels of physical activity in order to perform the tasks of daily living: shopping, housekeeping, yard work, and climbing stairs, for example. Cardiac rehabilitation programs teach people how to monitor exercise intensity, and how to feel safe and confident performing daily activity.

Regular physical activity leads to enormous health benefits when performed at levels prescribed by a cardiologist. With aerobic exercise, the heart becomes a more efficient pump, so it does not have to work as hard to perform a given amount of work. People are able to do more with less effort, which makes daily activities feel easier. Exercises to strengthen muscles and joints reduce the stress imposed by physical activities. Regular physical activity helps improve blood fat levels, blood sugar regulation, and blood pressure.

Slowing or even reversing the progression of heart disease usually entails changing other habits as well. Smokers must do all they can to quit. Dietary changes can help reduce harmful levels of blood fats and help control

blood sugar and blood pressure. Diet and exercise work together to help control weight. Medications are often prescribed to help control cardiovascular risk factors such as high blood pressure and diabetes.

My dad said the best thing about exercising after his heart surgery was that it helped him feel less worried and stressed.

The psychological benefits of physical activity may be the most important of all! Exercise reduces feelings of anxiety and depression, increases energy level, and improves mood. You sleep better, eat better, and feel better. Feeling better in turn helps you quit smoking, eat better, and stick to your cardiac rehabilitation lifestyle change program.

What kind of exercise is best?

Exercise recommendations must be individually tailored, since they depend on each patient's health and abilities. Exercise can be harmful for some heart conditions, so a cardiologist's guidance is essential. In general, exercise recommendations will be based on the results of an exercise stress test, which will help guide the cardiologist in his or her recommendations.

My mother just had bypass surgery. How can I help her find a good cardiac rehabilitation program?

Ask her cardiologist for guidance. Many patients feel pretty overwhelmed after surgery, and appreciate support getting back on their feet. Your help in interpreting the doctor's recommendations regarding your mother's rehabilitation program can make a big difference. Be sure you understand the doctor's recommendations, and be persistent with any questions you and your mother have. Your mother's doctor should be able to recommend what kind of a program is best for her, where you can find such a program, and whether or not your insurance will help pay for it.

Coming back after a heart attack, heart surgery, or a diagnosis of heart disease is a challenge. But exercise helps people with heart disease overcome the fear of exertion, and gives them confidence in performing the physical activities that are a part of daily life. Exercise not only improves physical function, but it helps people with heart disease become active participants in their recovery, and in life.

Exercise Improves Quality of Life for People With Cancer

"You want me to do what?" Many people with cancer are surprised to hear that exercise might help them feel better. Until recently, physicians advised their patients with cancer to rest, and avoid all activities that could worsen fatigue. This advice made sense. After all, fatigue is a message that your body needs rest. Exercising, it was thought, might deplete the body's limited energy supply.

Research has shown, however, that too much rest reduces the body's energy supply further. As muscles, joints, and bones become weaker, the activities required for daily living become increasingly difficult. A simple walk from the bedroom to the kitchen gets harder and harder. The solution? When possible, people with chronic illnesses such as cancer are advised to engage in mild to moderate physical activity to increase strength, endurance, and energy.

Should I check with my doctor first?

Yes. Each person is different, and you want to be sure exercise will be beneficial for you. Consider not only limitations imposed by illness, but also factors such as knee problems, back problems, and other health issues that would affect exercise recommendations. Get as much advice as possible, and ask what activities you can and cannot do.

If you have had surgery recently, or are undergoing bone marrow transplants, chemotherapy, or radiation treatments, you will want to get very specific guidelines. For example, you may not be able to exercise for a day or two following some types of chemotherapy, and not until symptoms such as nausea subside.

Not everyone with cancer should exercise, and there may be periods during treatment when rest is best. Ask your doctor about warning signs that indicate you should not exercise, such as fever or increased pain or swelling.

What kind of benefits can I expect if I exercise?

If your doctor has said you may exercise, it is important to begin very slowly and to progress very gradually. Research has shown that even very small amounts of activity, such as walking a few minutes several times a day, can help to reduce feelings of fatigue, and increase daily energy level. Physical activity may also improve sleep quality and help counteract insomnia.

As your muscles and joints become stronger, and as your endurance improves, daily tasks will begin to feel a little easier. If your treatments have led to muscle loss, exercise will help you regain some of your lost strength. Some people have found that participation in physical activity reduces feelings of stress, anxiety, and depression. Many report that exercise helps them feel better, more self-confident, and more in control of their treatment. Some people with cancer report that exercise helps them tolerate their treatments better.

What kind of exercise is best for people with cancer?

Cancer refers to over one hundred different diseases, each with its own characteristics and recommended treatments. No two people with cancer are alike, and research on exercise benefits for people with cancer is still fairly new. Thus, at this point in time there are no standard recommendations, except to start slowly and progress gradually to avoid injury.

If you have had surgery recently, you are probably working with a physical therapist to stretch and strengthen the muscles around the site of the surgery. You may also be walking short distances to build up your endurance.

As recovery progresses, you may be able to gradually add more exercise to your life. Work with a physical therapist or fitness professional who has experience working with people with cancer. You may even be able to locate an exercise group specifically for people with cancer in your area.

Exercise will improve your physical fitness if you ask your body to do just a little more than usual. So, for example, if you can walk for five minutes without getting tired, walk for six. If you already walk a mile or more, pick up the pace or walk a longer distance.

Most exercise programs include three types of activity. Aerobic activity, such as walking, cycling, or swimming, improves endurance. Strength training, such as calisthenics or weight lifting, increases the strength of muscles and joints. Stretching improves flexibility.

Mind Matters:
Can Lifestyle Prevent Memory Loss?

Some things improve with age, while others do not. Most older adults agree that memory belongs to the latter category. Researchers have begun to investigate, however, whether an age-related decline in memory is inevitable. Some believe that memory is a little bit like muscle. While some changes appear to occur with aging, no matter what we do, much of the loss can be slowed by a variety of healthful practices. And it seems that, like muscle, memory can be strengthened by appropriate exercise. Following are some suggestions for a "brain healthy" lifestyle.

Enjoy plenty of physical activity.

The brain has a rich circulatory system that supplies it with oxygen and nutrients, and removes wastes. Exercise improves the health of all of the arteries in the body by helping to prevent high blood pressure, and by improving blood sugar regulation and blood fat and cholesterol levels. Regular exercise reduces the likelihood that blood clots will form in the arteries, which could lead to stroke, an interruption of blood flow to the brain.

Physical activity may also prevent memory loss by reducing feelings of stress, anxiety, and depression. High levels of chronic stress are associated with the loss of nerve cells in regions of the brain important to memory. Depression, anxiety, and stress hinder memory in other ways as well, by interfering with the ability to concentrate. Our memories don't work well when we are distracted and unable to focus on the material we are supposed to remember.

Eat a heart-healthy diet.

The dietary practices that have been linked to heart health have also been associated with good mental performance. A Mediterranean-style diet with plenty of fruits, vegetables, whole grains, and legumes is best. While small amounts of meat and cheese can be included, intake of saturated and hydrogenated fats is generally low, and olive oil provides the principle source of fats. Nuts and fish, good sources of the omega-3 fats that reduce inflammation, should be consumed regularly.

Many nutrients have been recommended for slowing the aging process, although links between supplementation and brain health are lacking. We do know that nutritious diets high in plant foods are helpful, perhaps in part because they provide many of the antioxidant nutrients such as vitamins C and A. The phytochemicals abundant in plant foods may also retard the aging process.

An adequate intake of the B vitamin folate prevents high levels of homocysteine, a chemical found in the blood whose level is associated with increased risk of both artery disease and Alzheimer's disease. Adults need at least 400 micrograms of folate a day. Older adults whose diets are not always good may benefit from a daily multivitamin supplement. Nutrient deficiencies, especially of the B vitamins, contribute to memory problems in older adults.

Manage chronic health conditions, but watch for medication side effects.

Follow your physician's lifestyle and medication recommendations for diabetes, high blood pressure, high cholesterol, and depression. All of these can accelerate the aging of the arteries and contribute to memory loss over time. People on medications who experience a change in memory should check with their doctors to see whether this change could result from a medication side effect, in which case medications can be changed, or dosages adjusted.

Avoid tobacco products, and limit alcohol.

Tobacco products damage the arteries and other parts of your body in many ways. While a little alcohol appears to be protective for arteries and may help to prevent stroke, even low levels of alcohol consumption are associated with the loss of brain cells. We don't really know yet how much (if any) alcohol is safe when it comes to brain health.

Exercise your brain.

Challenging your brain improves the functioning of and builds connections among brain cells. Several studies have found a lower risk of Alzheimer's in people who engage in mentally stimulating activities. The better your brain development, the longer it will take for aging to result in mental deficits. Read, do puzzles, take classes; engage in plenty of creative and challenging work.

Nurture your emotional health.

Get enough sleep, relaxation, and recreation. Cultivate a positive outlook, nurture your spiritual growth, and make time for friends. Good emotional health nourishes your brain as well as your heart and soul.

90 Osteoporosis Prevention: What Kind of Exercise Is Best for Bones?

When you are young, your bones are just sort of there, and not the first thing you think about when considering your well-being. But many people become concerned about their bone strength when they reach midlife. This is especially true if osteoporosis runs in their families, or if they are at increased risk for osteoporosis because of other factors, such as medication use, poor nutrition, sedentary lifestyle, small size, smoking history, age, or Northern European or Asian descent.

Bones like to work hard. The worst thing for bones is a zero gravity environment; second worst is bed rest. A sedentary lifestyle is not so great either. Bones follow the "use it, or lose it" philosophy so common in the natural world.

Bones respond to force placed upon them by laying down more mineral and strengthening their structure to accommodate increased loading. Thinking about the forces produced by physical activities help us understand what kinds of exercise cause the greatest adaptation in, and greatest strengthening of bone tissue.

Exercise That Doesn't Cause Injury

Since inactivity causes bone mineral loss, your number one job is to avoid injury and illness that could interfere with physical activity. This means even if high-impact activities, such as jogging, increase bone strength, you should ignore this recommendation if jogging worsens or causes problems for you. Check with your health-care provider if you have any health concerns. A personal trainer can help you increase your exercise program slowly and gradually and help you avoid sports injuries.

Fortunately, in the long run, exercise generally helps prevent injury, especially if it improves strength and balance. Research has shown that regular physical activity can help to prevent falls, which can lead to fracture. It is especially interesting that regular physical activity reduces risk of bone fracture with a fall, even when no change in bone mineral density occurs. Regular physical activity seems to improve bone strength, even with no increase in mineral deposition.

If testing shows you are at very high risk for or have already developed osteoporosis, you may also need medications to help increase bone strength. Sometimes exercise and diet are not enough to prevent or treat osteoporosis.

Weight-Bearing Exercise

Exercise causes the greatest increase in bone strength when mechanical force is placed on bones, causing a deformation of bone cells. This force appears to be the signal that tells bones they need to get stronger. Weight-bearing activities such as tai chi, walking, jogging, running sports, and weight lifting place more force on the bones than weight-supported activities such as cycling and swimming.

Dynamic Exercise

Activities that produce constantly changing forces result in more strength improvement than continuous force. Walking and running, with the striking of the foot on the ground alternating with cessation of force, are examples of dynamic exercise, when talking about bones. Cross-country skiing, rowing, and machines such as elliptical trainers generally do not deliver large changes in force. While these activities provide terrific cardiovascular stimulation, they do not have as great an impact on bone strength. Similarly, wearing a weighted vest to perform low-intensity activity does not provide much bone stimulation. Jumping in a weighted vest, however, exerts a great deal of bone stimulation.

Relatively High-Impact and High-Intensity Exercise

Lifting heavy weights causes more bone adaptation than lifting lighter weights. Running exerts greater force than walking. Jumping, hopping, and skipping provide more impact than running.

Many sport activities provide good bone stimulation. Sport activities often combine running with jumping, and hitting and handling balls, so you get additional impact beyond running, as with soccer, basketball, and volleyball. Racquet sports provide impact in many ways. Handball is great, since you receive impact with both hands, and plenty of hard running.

High-impact aerobics classes often include jumping moves in many directions. Step aerobics and running stairs also provide good impact. Plyometric training incorporates very high impact work of variable directions and resistances.

What if these high impact activities are out of reach for you? Simply increasing walking pace increases the force your body receives as you take steps. So if you can walk, walk a little faster. If you can walk fast, add a few steps of slow jogging. Take the stairs more quickly. Add heavier weight to your workouts as you are able.

Bones need a healthy environment

To build bone strength you must consume adequate calories and protein, and enough calcium, potassium, magnesium, and vitamins D and K. Plenty of fruits and vegetables provide good nutrition and help build a good environment for bone growth. Avoid smoking, excessive alcohol, and excessive protein intake. Limit salt and empty calories.

Out of Shape? Or Exercise-Induced Asthma?

You go for a jog with your friends, but you find yourself out of breath while they are still able to carry on their conversation. Or maybe you have been working out for several weeks, but just don't seem to make much progress on the aerobic equipment. Endurance exercise feels really hard, and you wonder how so many of your friends seem to enjoy working out. Are you simply out of shape?

You may have exercise-induced asthma (EIA). Up to one in five people without chronic asthma experience asthma-like symptoms during or immediately following exercise. People often fail to realize they have EIA because the symptoms mimic the normal fatigue and breathlessness associated with intense exercise.

What are the symptoms of exercise-induced asthma?

The most common symptoms of EIA include the following. These may be experienced either during or after exercise, or both:

- Shortness of breath—you may still feel breathless up to 10 minutes after exercise
- Chest tightness
- Excess mucus production during exercise
- Wheezing, a whistling or rasping sound during breathing
- Cough, feeling a need to clear your airways

Less common symptoms include:

- Excessive fatigue with exercise, feeling out of shape at workloads that should not elicit such fatigue
- Lower performance than would be expected with current training levels
- Sore throat with exercise
- Headache
- Stomach cramps

How can I tell if I have EIA, or am just out of shape?

Your health-care provider can give you a lung function test with an instrument called a spirometer. A spirometer can measure how much air you are able to forcefully exhale in one second. You can take this simple test at rest, and then again after some kind of breathing challenge, such as fast breathing or an exercise test. If your post-challenge value is significantly (usually 10 percent or more) lower than your resting value, exercise-induced asthma is diagnosed.

How is EIA different from regular asthma?

Some researchers believe that EIA (or they might call it exercise-induced bronchoconstriction) does not always involve as much inflammation as other forms of asthma. But others believe it's all the same, just different triggers.

About 90 percent of people who experience chronic asthma find that exercise also triggers asthma attacks. Many people with EIA have other allergic conditions such as allergies or hay fever. Everyone agrees that people should be treated on an individual basis, according to the severity of their symptoms and which triggers provoke asthma symptoms.

Is EIA less serious than other types of asthma?

Any condition that causes difficulty breathing should be taken seriously. Although most asthma attacks respond well to medication, every year many people are rushed to the hospital with breathing difficulties resulting from asthma. Some people, including athletes, even die from asthma. Almost 5,000 asthma deaths occur in the United States each year.

Why does exercise cause asthma symptoms?

No one knows exactly why exercise triggers asthma symptoms. Some researchers believe it has to do with the changes in the airways that occur with heavy breathing. Normally, the nose humidifies and warms the inhaled air before it reaches your airways. As exercise becomes more intense, you breathe through your mouth instead of through your nose. Large volumes of dry, cool air draw moisture from the airways. As the airways lose moisture, chemical changes in the cells may trigger the allergic reactions associated with asthma.

How is EIA treated?

A variety of asthma medications help prevent symptoms. These medications must be prescribed by your doctor. People with EIA must work closely with their providers to be sure their symptoms are adequately controlled.

People with allergies may be able to avoid conditions that exacerbate their asthma. For example, people allergic to pollen may have less EIA when they exercise indoors during pollen season.

Many people with asthma find that respiratory infections (colds, flu) trigger asthma symptoms. You may need to avoid intense or endurance exercise when you are sick.

Some types of exercise may be easier for you. Stop and start activities, such as team sports and racquet sports, may be less problematic. Exercise in cold, dry air tends to be more challenging, although wearing a facemask designed for cold-weather exercise may reduce breathing discomfort. Swimming in a warm, humid environment is comfortable for many people with EIA.

Exercising With Asthma

Over the past 30 years athletes with asthma have competed successfully in all types of sporting events. They have served as inspiring examples to all people with asthma, young and old, that this condition need not be a barrier to athletic excellence.

This is remarkable because physical activity can be a potent asthma trigger. Not so long ago, children with asthma were told to stay out of physical education class, and adults avoided any excess exertion that might bring on an attack.

Fortunately, times have changed, and the treatment of asthma has improved considerably. People with asthma are still told to avoid those things that trigger an asthma response, with one important exception: exercise.

What is asthma?

An asthma attack is characterized by wheezing, chest tightness and burning, and shortness of breath. Something triggers the smooth muscle lining the lungs to contract, and this restricts the flow of air into and out of the airways, making breathing difficult. The mucous membranes that line these airways become irritated and secrete excess mucous that may further restrict the flow of air.

Asthma can be triggered by allergens in the air, such as pollen, mold, feathers and animal dander. Cigarette smoke and other components of air pollution can initiate or worsen an asthmatic response. Some people get asthma from food allergies, upper respiratory tract infections and emotional stress. Cold, dry air will elicit an asthmatic response in susceptible people. So will exercise. Asthma that occurs in response to exercise is known as exercise-induced asthma, or EIA.

Asthma is a condition that affected people must learn to live with. There is no cure, so it is important to understand what triggers asthma for you, and make whatever adjustments you can so that it interferes with your activities as little as possible.

Is it possible to only get asthma from exercise?

Yes. Many people do not even realize they have EIA, since the symptoms of asthma mimic that out-of-breath, out-of-shape feeling that occurs during a demanding workout. EIA is suspected if the difficulty breathing continues for several minutes after exercise is over, and if it is worse when you exercise in cold, dry air. People with a history of allergies and hay fever may experience EIA during allergy season.

What's the best type of exercise for people with EIA?

EIA seems to be caused by the cooling and drying of airways that results from the increased breathing that occurs during exercise. Each breath of air is heated and humidified by your lungs, so as the volume of air that you are breathing increase, so does the loss of heat and moisture from your lungs. This may trigger an asthmatic response in sensitive people.

Therefore, the best exercise for people with EIA is that which minimizes water and heat loss. Swimming is ideal, since the air in the pool is both warm and moist. Indoor exercise is preferable to exercising outdoors in cold seasons and climates, or during allergy season.

Intermittent exercise is sometimes better tolerated than continuous activity. Short periods of exercise are interspersed with a minute or two of rest. Circuit weight training is an example of intermittent exercise.

Can exercise help prevent or reduce the severity of asthma?

Although exercise cannot prevent asthma, getting into shape can increase your tolerance for physical activity. Because your stamina improves, the flight of stairs that used to bring on wheezing and shortness of breath becomes less of a problem.

Wellness Through the Lifespan

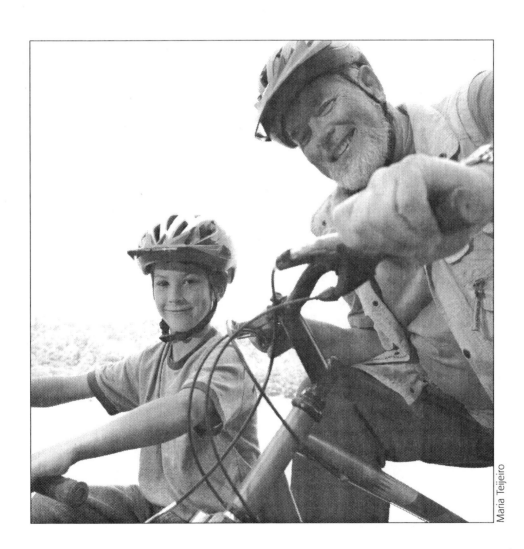

Maria Teijeiro

Chapter 8

Choosing a Sports Program for Your Child

The benefits of a good sports experience are many: positive self-esteem, regular physical activity, improvements in physical fitness, lower risk of depression and, best of all, lots of fun. But sport involvement also requires a great deal of commitment in terms of time and sometimes money. Participation in sports also carries some risk of injury, even in the safest programs.

Parents play a critical role in determining whether their children get involved in sports programs. Your children are more likely to participate if you value sport experience and have a positive attitude about youth sports programs. Parents are also usually the ones who provide the money and transportation required to be part of a sports program. You may need to help your children shop for equipment, and get to practice and competitions on time. Many parents even spend time practicing sports skills with their children at home.

Parents also help to determine the nature of their child's sports experience. Parents can create enjoyable experiences by signing their children up for programs that will be fun. They can also create stress and anxiety by placing excessive pressure on their children to excel, or enrolling them in programs that are unsuitably demanding. Following are a few suggestions for helping your children have positive sports experiences.

Think long term.

What are your reasons for encouraging sports involvement? Most parents hope that sports will improve their child's physical and emotional health and development. They want sports to be challenging yet fun, so that their children can feel successful and proud of their progress.

The best sports experiences develop when children and programs are a good match. Look for programs that are appropriate for your child's age, motor development, and interests. Young children need experiences that teach skills through games and play, with less emphasis on competition. Older children may be ready for more competitive experiences, although many will still prefer something low-key.

A child's early sports experiences are important, because if these experiences are embarrassing or discouraging, children (and adults!) may decide they hate sports and stay away from them forever. This is unfortunate. Many children who have been pushed (too hard?) to participate in sports at a young age drop out before they reach adolescence. Yet the teenage years are the time when boys and girls really need sports and other forms of vigorous physical activity to help them deal with the emotional stress of their changing bodies and moods. When you think long term, you look for sports programs that are most likely to give your child a positive emotional experience.

Talk to other families involved in youth sport programs in your area. As you ask around about good coaches and programs, you will start to hear certain names over and over again. Ask kids and their parents why they chose the program, and what they like about it. Are these the qualities you think your child would enjoy?

Make safety a priority.

Be sure your children have the proper safety equipment recommended for their sports, and that the equipment fits well and is in good condition. Encourage children to drink plenty of water before and during practice and competition, and to avoid vigorous exertion if the weather is hot and humid. Attend to aches and pains that could be an early sign of overuse injury. Ask the coach to limit your child's participation if injuries develop.

Show positive support, and model good sportsmanship.

Show an interest in your child's sports experience, but find a level of involvement that works for you and your children. Be supportive, but don't dominate the experience. If you are unable to attend a game, ask your child about it. Monitor the experiences your children are having. Are things going well? Do they like going to practices and competitions?

Be a good spectator at contests. Sit where the coach asks you to sit, and cheer all the children on your team, not just your child. Never boo the opposing team (these are just kids!). Don't try to coach from the sidelines, or argue with the coach or referees. And be sure to thank the coaches for their work.

Strength Training for Kids: Safety First

Weight rooms and gyms used to be thought of as the domain of big, burly guys, who moved confidently through their workouts, sweat glistening and muscles bulging. As medical researchers began to discover the many health benefits of strength training, ordinary adults began to infiltrate this mysterious domain. Even women began learning to use strength-training equipment. Even the very old have begun visiting the weight room to combat frailty and weakness. What's next? Kids?

The idea of kids in weight rooms may seem odd at first. But recent research suggests that age-appropriate strength-training programs have a lot to offer children and adolescents in terms of health, fitness, and fun. If you are thinking about strength-training exercise for the children and adolescents in your life, the following are a few things to consider.

Strength training exercise should be supervised.

Injuries are most common in home gyms in children playing around with equipment. Weight equipment can be heavy and dangerous. Serious injury can result when equipment is used in inappropriate ways, such as when people lift weights that are much too heavy or drop equipment on themselves or others.

Strength training should be incorporated into a lifestyle that includes plenty of physical activity.

Strength training is not a substitute for games, sports, or outdoor recreation. Children and adolescents need to walk, hike, swim, and ride bicycles. Children need active play. They need good physical education programs in school.

Strength training sessions should be taught by a knowledgeable, adult instructor.

Be sure the instructor understands the special needs of children and adolescents, and is able to communicate well to the age group involved. A low student-to-instructor ratio is best, especially for beginners.

Programs should be noncompetitive and fun.

Injuries can occur when students compete to see who can lift the most weight, and they lift inappropriately heavy loads, straining joints and muscles. Programs are safer when students track their own progress rather than compare themselves to others. Programs must be fun, or children lose interest quickly, or acquire a dislike for strength training, a dislike that may last for many years.

Children and adolescents should train for the right reasons.

Good reasons to participate in strength training are to increase strength, prevent injury, improve physical fitness and body composition, and improve sports performance. Some children and adolescents begin weight training hoping to achieve a superhero's physique. They are likely to become frustrated and disappointed, and in extreme cases to develop an obsession with how they look, and even eating disorders.

Programs should begin slowly and increase training demands gradually.

This is true for any exercise program at any age. A strength-training program should be individually designed for each child. Early lessons should focus primarily on safety and technique, using a light and easily managed resistance.

Strength-training equipment should be appropriate for the age group.

Strength-training equipment should fit the child. Younger children may not fit into station machines built for adults. Exercise should not be attempted if this is the case, because the body may not be properly supported, and exercise will not be very effective. Programs for children often rely on free weights (dumb bells and bar bells), rubber tubing, and calisthenics such as abdominal curls.

As strength increases, resistance is usually increased as well, to encourage continued fitness benefits. Injury may result, however, if too much increase is applied too soon. An increase of only 5 to 10 percent is recommended; this small increase may be impossible with many station machines. A good program is driven by the user's fitness level and exercise needs, not by the type of equipment available.

Children must be old enough to listen carefully and follow directions.

The exact age at which children can do this varies, so check with the instructor to see whether the young child is really ready for the program.

95 Positive Lifestyle Change for Your Overweight Son or Daughter

Today's environment features the ready availability of tasty food, much of it too high in sugar, fat, salt and calories, and too few opportunities for physical activity. We eat too much and exercise too little. The result is obesity: too much body fat, and the health problems that often follow. Health professionals have expressed alarm at the rising obesity rates in all segments of the population, including children and adolescents.

Not every overweight child becomes an overweight adult. Many children "grow out of" obesity at some point. And many children who are thin or normal weight will become obese during their adult years. Helping children develop healthful lifestyles that include good food choices, lots of love, and plenty of physical activity prevents obesity, gives overweight kids a chance to "grow out of" their obesity, and provides kids with the skills they need to nurture good health throughout their lives.

If you have overweight children, you have an extra incentive to take a good look at your family's routine. Fortunately, the positive changes you make for your overweight children benefit everyone in your family. With good nutrition and plenty of physical activity you and everyone in your family reduce risk of developing health problems such as high blood pressure and type 2 diabetes.

Is My Child Overweight?

If you think your child is overweight, check with his or her health-care provider. Obesity is determined by checking your child's weight against the weight of other children his or her age and sex. Some parents see their children as fat even though they are of normal weight, while others overlook obesity problems. (It's just a little baby fat; he'll grow out of it.) Both create problems.

If your provider finds that your child is overweight, he or she can give you more information on making positive lifestyle changes. In many cases, simple changes can help your child achieve a more normal weight as time goes by. In other cases, your provider may refer you to a more aggressive weight loss program, especially if your child is already developing obesity-related health problems. Either way, you will be encouraged to provide nutritious meals and snacks, to limit junk food, and to increase family activity levels.

Assess the Situation

Take a look at your children's and your family's lifestyle. Try to uncover the reasons your child is overweight. Too much snacking? Television? Does your child eat in response to stress? Once you figure out the cause, you can begin to find solutions.

Dieting Versus Positive Lifestyle

Restrictive, rigid diets are very harmful to children for many reasons. First, they are usually stressful and create bad feelings. Children (and adults) who feel bad resent the changes in their diets. And many people overeat when they feel bad! Food cravings may develop in response to dietary restriction and increase the drive to overeat.

Restrictive dieting may not provide adequate nutrition. Good nutrition is especially important for growing bodies. Children and teens who diet may compromise bone density and growth. They may lack the energy and motivation to do well in school.

Restrictive diets that focus on quick weight loss can lead to a focus on weight loss, rather than health. A focus on weight loss in turn can lead to other quick weight loss strategies, such as use of diet pills and supplements, cigarette smoking, laxative abuse, and other harmful behaviors.

Lastly, restrictive diets don't usually work. People don't learn how to make good food choices, and how to live with readily available food without gaining weight. When people fail on their diets they feel guilty and bad about themselves. Ironically, dieting can even cause weight gain when people overeat in response to dieting stress and feel that it's not worth even trying to lose weight because they will only fail.

Instead of restrictive dieting, limit empty calories. In one study, teens lost about a pound a week simply by drinking water instead of soft drinks. Help your children learn to eat in response in hunger rather than boredom or discomfort.

Physical Activity

Many overweight children and teens avoid physical activity because it's uncomfortable or feels awkward. They may be slower than their classmates, and feel embarrassed in exercise clothes. Overweight kids may be chosen last for teams, teased, or bullied.

Be persistent as you help your children find opportunities for physical activity. Walk or bike for transportation, exercise at home with videotapes, and look for individualized fitness programs at your local fitness center. Look for coaches and instructors who have a good attitude and make your child or teen feel good.

HANDOUT 96 Feeding Your Children: Good Nutrition for Healthy Futures

Good nutrition during childhood helps support optimal growth and development. It can also reduce risk for chronic diseases, such as type 2 diabetes, high blood pressure, and heart disease later in life. Good eating habits and food choices, along with plenty of physical activity help kids to maintain a healthy body weight and prevent obesity.

Once kids reach adolescence, they often buy their food away from home. Therefore, the childhood years, especially through age 12, are parents' best chance to exert a meaningful influence over their children's food choices. During this time children are a relatively captive audience when it comes to mealtime, as parents and caregivers still purchase and prepare most of the food. Once children enter elementary school, they are old enough to begin to learn about nutrition basics. This is a receptive time for learning because children in grades one through six are fairly cooperative and still generally like and respect their parents (which is not always true of adolescents!).

Basic Guidelines

Good nutrition for children age 6 to 12 is quite similar to good nutrition for adults: children need to eat a variety of foods from different food categories. You can use the Food Guide Pyramid as a guide, aiming to give children the minimum number of servings in each category most days. This means at least two servings of fruit, three servings of vegetables, two servings of dairy, two servings of proteins foods (meat, fish, eggs, peanut butter or beans), and several servings of grains and grain products. Within each group, try to select a variety of foods, and look for foods that are high in vitamins and minerals while low in sugar and salt.

In general, parents and caregivers need to help children to replace empty calorie foods such as soda and candy with fruits, vegetables, and whole grains. Occasional treats are fine, but these should supplement, not replace, a well-rounded diet. Many treats and snacks can be nourishing as well as delicious.

Simple Changes

Simple changes introduced gradually with love and some nutrition education work best for most families. Parents should begin with a survey of their own eating habits and home food environment. What kinds of foods are on hand? What are the snack choices? A parent's own good example of a healthy relationship with nutritious food helps children internalize healthful behavior and attitudes. Following are some suggestions for simple changes that can improve your family's eating habits.

Increase the variety of fruit you have on hand for snacks and meals.

Children generally like fruit, so increasing fruit intake is fairly simple. Reach for fresh, frozen, or canned. If using canned fruits, choose low-sugar varieties. Try for a variety of colors throughout the day, such as blueberries on breakfast cereal, peaches with lunch, and a banana for a snack. Especially nutritious are watermelon, cantaloupe, citrus fruits, and berries.

Serve the vegetables your children like best often.

Children generally like blander vegetables such as potatoes, corn, and carrots, but every child is different, so cater to yours!

Ask children to try just one bite of all foods at mealtime.

Taking just one or two bites is not too much to ask. As children try new foods, even ones they don't like, they get used to new tastes. That one bite works best at the beginning of the meal when the child is still hungry. Since mealtimes should be pleasant and cheerful, this "one bite" should not be a punishment, but just something you do.

Serve small portions of a variety of foods.

Serving small portions prevents your child from filling up on a favorite food, such as noodles or bread. Small portions also increase the likelihood that less food will be wasted. Children (and adults) should stop eating when they feel full. Asking children to keep eating until they "clean their plate" is now thought to be training for future obesity. Learning to listen to hunger and satiety signals helps prevent obesity.

Sneak vegetables into snacks and meals.

Disguise vegetables with sauces and dips. Add broccoli or spinach to tomato sauce over noodles. Crunchy vegetable sticks taste great with bean dip or hummus.

Look for creative ways to replace empty-calorie foods.

Instead of soft drinks, try mixing equal parts of fruit juice and seltzer to make spritzers. Make your own whole-grain pancakes with added wheat germ, bran, or ground flaxseed.

Should Children and Teens Use Sports Supplements?

Most coaches and parents have noticed the growing number of products marketed to athletes and exercisers, products claiming to increase energy or trim body fat. No longer found only in "health food" stores, these products now adorn the shelves of supermarkets and drug stores as well. All sorts of products, including some very questionable supplements, are sold over the Internet. The promises sound good, and appeal to consumers of all ages.

Although some of these products can be helpful, coaches and parents of young people should keep an eye on what is going into the bodies of the children and adolescents in their care. Coaches and parents must teach young athletes to be informed consumers, and help them navigate the dietary supplement marketplace.

Marketing and labels for these products are often misleading and deceptive.

Young people tend to assume supplements are regulated the same way as drugs. They figure if the supplement is on the shelves, it must be safe. But dietary supplements are not regulated as stringently as drugs. The labels and marketing materials for these products may be quite misleading. Children and teens may not read the find print but focus instead on the picture of the body builder and the implied messages on the label.

Dietary supplements may contain unlisted ingredients.

Dietary supplements sometimes contain substances not listed on the label. This can occur either from carelessness of the manufacturer or because the manufacturer intentionally adds unlisted products to enhance the efficacy of the preparation. Added caffeine, for example, may make the user think the product is "doing something." Very rarely, supplements may even be contaminated with ingredients that can cause severe illness, liver failure, and even death.

Young people may take high doses.

Young people may not use a product as directed. They may figure that since a product is "natural" it is safe at any level. Supplements are often safe when used as directed, but can have harmful effects at high doses. This is why so many people got into trouble with ephedra (adults as well as kids). A little is fine for most adults, but high doses can cause jitters, anxiety, and a rapid heart rate.

Some ingredients are not good for children or teens.

Some of the ingredients in supplements, especially those marketed as muscle building or sports recovery products, are potentially harmful to growing bodies. For example,

some supplements contain aspirin, which increases risk of Reyes syndrome, a rare but potentially fatal disorder, in children. Caffeine and other stimulants may cause anxiety and sleeplessness. The long-term effects of many supplement ingredients are unknown in children (or adults for that matter!).

Even ingredients considered to be "safe" for adults have not been tested in children.

Consider creatine, widely used by many high school athletes. While this supplement appears to be safe for adults, no studies have looked at its safety or efficacy in children or teens. The same is true for the prohormones, such as DHEA, or even high doses of single amino acids such as carnitine.

Safe use sometimes progresses to unsafe use.

Children and teens often fail to distinguish between fairly safe and potentially dangerous supplements. They may see little difference between a bodybuilding protein shake that is probably harmless or even helpful, and a drink that also contains prohormones and caffeine.

For some adolescents, the use of legal supplements may progress to the use of illegal supplements such as steroids or growth hormone. Researchers estimate that up to five to ten percent of high school males, and about two to three percent of high school females, experiment with steroids in a given school year. Steroids, in turn, sometimes become a "gateway drug" to the use of other illegal substances such as cocaine.

Educate your players and children about the products you endorse.

Explain what is in them and why they are helpful. You don't need to give up sports drinks or energy bars! Most children who play sports welcome a cold sports drink on a hot day during a practice or contest. They like the drinks because they taste good; coaches and parents like these drinks because they replenish fluids and prevent dehydration. The carbohydrate in these drinks also helps to keep blood sugar up and thus to delay fatigue. For endurance athletes, sports bars, goos, and gels may provide much needed energy when there is no time or appetite for real food.

Explain also why other products are discouraged. Explain how caffeine and other drugs can hurt performance in the long run by interfering with good health. Athletes of all ages should learn how to enhance health and performance with physical conditioning, good nutrition, and a balanced lifestyle.

98 Healthy Adolescents? Tips for Parents

Many parents call it the best of times and the worst of times: adolescence! It is a time of passion and emerging identity. Parents will also attest that special tact is required for guiding adolescents toward healthy lifestyles. In fact, many parents wonder whether there's anything they can do to help their sons and daughters acquire healthy habits during this time when parents feel they have limited influence.

Healthful eating habits and regular physical activity are important in childhood, adolescence and adulthood. They reduce a person's risk for many chronic diseases, such as obesity, heart disease, and high blood pressure later in life. Since these illnesses have no cure, we must focus on prevention beginning in childhood and continuing throughout our lives.

Physical activity is especially important for teens because it enhances mental health and increases resistance to the negative effects of the many stresses teens experience. It also improves body image and self-confidence. Some studies have even found a link between regular physical activity and academic performance.

Many adolescents remain quite active throughout their teenage years, but the majority become less active as they approach adulthood. How can you encourage your sedentary teen to become more active? Following are a few helpful hints from parents of teens and from teachers who have spent years working with adolescents.

Model healthful behaviors and attitudes.

Your diet and exercise attitudes and behaviors have been absorbed by your children throughout childhood. If you generally eat well-balanced meals, manage your stress and enjoy regular exercise, your children have a head start. And don't worry; you don't have to be perfect. Just do your best for the sake of your own health and that of your children. James A. Baldwin once said, "Children have never been very good at listening to their elders, but they have never failed to imitate them."

As much as possible, serve well-balanced meals at home, including plenty of fruits and vegetables. Keep healthful snack foods on hand. Encourage teens to be active for the right reasons: health, fitness, stress management and, most of all, fun. This is crucial since teens are often obsessed with weight control and appearance. While wanting to look good may motivate teens to follow healthy lifestyle recommendations, it can also strengthen an obsession with looks. This obsession can lead to preoccupations with eating and exercise that are often difficult to overcome.

Don't focus on weight loss.

Again, emphasize a healthful lifestyle. Focusing on weight sets your teen up for failure, since weight loss is difficult to achieve. Teens become easily discouraged and may give up quickly when expected results are not instantaneous (and the healthful kind of weight loss, fat loss, never is). When weight loss is the focus, people become angry and disappointed. Remember, your number-one goal is to help your teen and family survive the adolescent years with your loving relationships intact!

Encourage after-school and summer physical activity programs.

Let your teen enroll in after-school and summer camp physical activity programs. Find out what is available in your community. Check into after-school programs, community centers, YMCAs, sports programs, dance classes, and fitness centers. Some parents even start their own groups. Choose activities your teen is most excited about (or least resistant to). Then, sign your teens up with their friends.

Limit sedentary activities.

If your teen spends a lot of time watching television or movies, or playing video and computer games, work out a reasonable compromise.

Harness that adolescent idealism.

Many teens love to put their energy into service activities. Encourage your son or daughter to sign up for a walkathon or dance-a-thon that makes donations to a worthy cause.

Have the energy to parent your teenager.

Parenting a teen can be demanding. Extra stress can upset your own equilibrium, which is more important than ever during this period. Keep an optimistic perspective, and remember that adolescence doesn't last forever. Get professional help if parenting struggles are getting you down, or your teen is in trouble.

Female Athletes: Support Healthy Bones

Many women don't think about bone health until it's too late to do most of the things they were supposed to be doing in their teens, 20s and 30s. While it's never too late to make healthful changes in your lifestyle, the earlier you begin, the stronger and more beneficial the effects of those changes.

I thought osteoporosis wasn't a problem until middle age?

Young women should be concerned about bone health because it is during their teens, 20s and 30s that bone mass is built. By the late 30s, bone mass begins to decline. The decline accelerates after menopause, which usually occurs somewhere between the ages of 45 and 55.

While osteoporosis usually does not develop until middle age or older, it can also occur in young women who have stopped (or never started) having menstrual periods. In several studies, such women in their 20s were found to have the bone density characteristics of women in their 70s, and the types of fractures and rounded back posture that go with it. This type of damage is often painful and irreversible. Young women who have sustained vertebral fractures will never have youthful spines again, even if their menstrual cycles resume.

Osteoporosis is not the only reason to be concerned about bone health. Female athletes with low-density bones are vulnerable to sports injuries such as stress fractures. Such injuries can short-circuit their athletic development, and even put an end to participation in their favorite activities.

What can I do to build healthy bones?

The most important way to build healthy bones is to maintain a healthy lifestyle. A nutritious diet, moderate exercise, not smoking and limiting alcohol intake can all help you build healthy bones. If you experience menstrual irregularity, be sure to see your doctor to determine the cause and appropriate treatment. A regular cycle is especially important because it generates estrogen, a female hormone that helps protect against loss of bone mineral.

I know calcium intake is important. How else is diet important?

Frequent dieting contributes to osteoporosis, especially if diets are very restrictive and contain fewer than 1,600 calories a day. Not only do very-low-calorie diets fail to supply calcium, they also give the body the message that starvation is near at hand. Such a message causes metabolic changes, including a drop in metabolic rate and, for young women, irregular menstrual cycles. Very-low-calorie diets are rarely effective weight-control techniques, anyway. You are better off developing healthful eating habits you can live with for a lifetime. Regular exercise is also essential for lifelong weight control.

How can I tell if I am losing bone density?

Ask your doctor. Bone density measurements are becoming more widely available, and your doctor may know of a health center that performs them. You can probably figure out from your health history (exercise, diet, menstrual cycle) whether bone density could become a problem for you. Our bones are easy to ignore since we can't see them, but you certainly do not want to wait until stress fractures or spinal curvature develops before you begin to do something.

Many people overestimate the importance of having low body fat for their sport. Athletes who fight to maintain a body fat below what is a healthy level for them are fighting nature and harming themselves in the process. While it may seem worth the sacrifice, don't lose sight of your long-term health and fitness. Your running days will be numbered unless you maintain good health. Many women find that reducing their exercise volume by about 10 percent and putting on just a few pounds is enough to cause the resumption of their menstrual cycles without sacrificing their competitive shape. In fact, many women find performance improves, and they overcome staleness with these changes, since they become healthier and have more energy.

100 Preventing College Weight Gain

Starting college means many changes, especially if it means moving away from home. A new environment and a new schedule require you to form new habits. Many students fall into new patterns of eating and working that lead to unnecessary and unwanted weight gain, not to mention fatigue, stress, anxiety and poor academic performance. But preventing college weight gain is not difficult; it just takes a little bit of planning. Best of all, the habits that help you maintain a healthy weight will also help you feel alert and energized, as well as do your best in school.

Schedule physical activity into your semester.

It's easy to say you will get to the fitness center regularly, but good intentions often fall by the wayside once assignments begin to pile up. Instead, schedule a physical education, dance or recreation course into your schedule. Take an activity you enjoy, or try something new.

If you are on a sports team, you will automatically make time to train and compete. You will also learn how to manage your time to get everything done! When your season ends, be sure you make a plan for remaining active in your off-season.

Check out active extracurricular activities, like your campus outing club. Go dancing, sign up for intramural activities or start your own walking group. Make exercise an important part of your semester schedule, and remember that your health is a priority.

Get enough sleep.

While a few short nights won't kill you, regular sleep helps you complete more work of a higher quality in a shorter period of time, so you actually spend less time studying, but get better results. Getting enough sleep prevents fatigue and improves health, which will make you more resistant to the next cold that hits campus. Fatigue can also lead to feelings of hunger, so you'll be less likely to overeat if you get enough sleep.

Many students find that too much caffeine interferes with sleep quality. Drinking several cups of coffee, tea or soda may seem like a helpful study aid late at night when you have a lot of work to complete. But if poor sleep results, you will fall behind the next day.

Deal with stress.

Don't let your problems pile up. Try to stay caught up with your assignments, and get help if you find the work difficult or are falling behind. Talk to a counselor if you experience difficulties adjusting to college. Make time to have fun with your new friends.

Regular physical activity reduces feelings of stress, anxiety and depression. Sticking to your exercise plans will not only prevent weight gain, but it will help you feel good, too.

Eat well-balanced meals, and avoid excessive snacking.

Eating out is a great way to gain weight! If you eat in an all-you-can-eat dining hall, scan the selection before each meal and decide what you want the most. Fill your plate with plenty of fruits and vegetables, and limit junk food. Make conscious choices instead of trying one of everything. Eat slowly, enjoy your food, and stop eating when you start to feel full.

Eat breakfast. Breakfast helps your brain wake up so you will get the most from your classes; it also keeps you from overeating later in the day. If you are not hungry when you first awaken, take a snack with you to eat later in the morning.

If you don't know much about food, take a nutrition course at your college. Learn which foods give you good nutrition and which are not worth the calories.

Don't diet.

Dieters are more apt to gain weight in the long run. Students need fuel to support their high-energy lifestyles. If you need to lose weight, gradually reduce the junk foods in your diet. Eat regular, small meals and healthy snacks. Study in the library where you will be less tempted to snack while you work. Get plenty of exercise, and get involved in interesting activities that keep you away from food.

101 The Student Body: Make Exercise Part of Your Student Schedule

Success in high school and college depends on the ability to comprehend large volumes of difficult material. Comprehension, in turn, requires that you focus with alert attention on what you are hearing and reading, your memory in high gear, all the wheels turning. Academic success is more often associated with mental workouts rather than a trip to the gym. But did you know that regular physical activity can boost your brainpower and academic productivity? Exercise has other great benefits, too.

Regular physical activity helps reduce feelings of stress.

School tends to be a high stress environment. Stress is the ultimate distraction, and the most common reason that students fail in their classes. It's hard to concentrate when you are distracted by problems. Obviously, exercise will not make problems go away! You must still deal with your financial difficulties, relationship issues, and whatever else is causing you stress. But a good workout helps stop the worrying, anxiety, and depression that easily become part of the stress package. Regular exercise improves your brain chemistry and relaxes your muscles, yet leaves you feeling focused and alert (without the caffeine jitters).

Exercise helps you sleep better.

Many students report improvement in sleep quality once they begin exercising regularly. Academic overload can lead to late night studying, too much caffeine, and feeling tired and wired when it's finally time to sleep. Noisy apartments and dormitories make sleep difficult as well. Exercise can't overcome all these problems: you will still need to quit procrastinating and drinking too much caffeine, but exercise can be part of your strategy for improving sleep quality, so you are alert and focused when it's time for homework and class.

Regular physical activity helps strengthen your immune system.

Spending so much time in close quarters with hundreds of people, especially people from around the world, increases your exposure germs. Students (and everyone working in such an environment!) must do all they can to stay healthy. One good cold can knock you out for a week or more, while the readings, papers, exams, and other assignments pile up.

Plenty of hand washing reduces the spread of germs. Adequate sleep, stress management, good nutrition, and regular exercise help to keep your immune system in good

shape. But be careful: getting *too much* exercise can reduce immunity. How much is too much? Anything that is way more than you are used to doing.

Should you exercise when you are sick? You are better off in bed: your body needs rest, not exercise, once you are sick. And why spread your germs around the fitness center?

Exercise helps prevent obesity.

Ever hear of the Freshman Fifteen? Days of sitting in class and studying in the library combined with cafeteria dining, fast food, and late night pizza often result in unwanted weight gain when students leave home for college. Obesity can also develop in high school.

Obesity prevention is simple in theory: exercise more, daily if possible, and eat less. Choose healthful, wholesome food, including plenty of fruits and vegetables, and limit the junk. Take a class in nutrition or health if you need more information on how to eat well (even on a budget).

Exercise will help you quit smoking.

Now's the time! The sooner you quit, the better you will feel. You are probably intending to quit someday, so do it now before the addiction gets worse. Smoking really screws up your brain chemistry, and the longer you smoke, the more depressed you will feel when you quit. Exercise will help you get through the withdrawal symptoms, and reduce risk of weight gain.

School is a great place to find activities you enjoy and make new friends.

Check out the options at your school for adding physical activity to your schedule. Take a physical education class for credit, or look for noncredit alternatives. Many colleges and high schools offer a variety of activities. Try a new sport, or return to an old favorite. Learn yoga, tai chi, or Pilates, or do aerobics for fun.

Join a team: you'll be forced to work out and manage your time. If you are not varsity material, check out club sports or intramurals. Want to get outdoors? Does your school offer outdoor adventure activities? Do you have an outing club? If not, start one with your friends!

Students on campuses usually have ideal conditions for active transportation: bike and walk whenever possible. You'll save money on gas, reduce pollution, and get exercise at the same time. Take the stairs at every opportunity to classes, offices, and dorm rooms.

Exercise Guidelines for a Healthy Pregnancy

Congratulations! You're expecting, and you've heard exercise can help you have a healthy pregnancy and a healthy baby. Following are some guidelines to help you make the most of your workouts during pregnancy.

- Be sure to check with your doctor before exercising during pregnancy. While exercise is recommended for most pregnant women, certain complications can occur which make exercise dangerous for you, the baby, or both of you.

- If you are new to exercise, choose low-impact activities such as walking, low-impact aerobics, and swimming. As your shape grows and changes, you will want to avoid activities that can throw you off balance or cause you to fall or be bumped (e.g., skiing or horseback riding).

- Prenatal exercise classes can lead you in exercises to strengthen pelvic, abdominal, and back muscles, which take much of the burden of pregnancy and childbirth. Your provider may also recommend exercises for these muscle groups.

- Regular exercise (at least three times a week) is safer than occasional exercise. When you exercise regularly, you body adapts in many ways. Occasional exercise is more likely to cause injury.

- Warm up before exercise, increasing exercise intensity gradually. A warm-up gives your body a chance to prepare for more vigorous exercise. At the end of your workout, slowly decrease intensity with a cool down.

- Drink water before, during, and after exercise to avoid dehydration. The amount of water you need will depend upon how hard you are exercising and on the temperature and humidity. In general, try to drink about 2 cups of water an hour before you exercise, and then a cup of water for every 20 minutes of exercise. Remember that you need to drink even though you may not be thirsty.

- Do not get overheated. Do not exercise if the weather is hot and humid, or if you have a fever. Heat stress may be harmful to the developing baby.

- Wear a good support bra and comfortable clothing. Good shoes appropriate for your activity will help protect against injury and help your feet carry a heavier load.

- Protect your back. Your growing belly changes your center of gravity in a way that puts more stress on your back. Try to use good posture and body mechanics. Avoid exercises or lifting in a bending over (rounded back) position.

- If you are lifting weight, use lighter weights (to avoid injuring your joints) and do not hold your breath. Remember that your joints are more flexible during pregnancy, and may thus be more prone to injury.

- Avoid exercises that are done lying on your back. The weight of the uterus presses on important blood vessels, which reduces blood flow to you and your baby.

- Eat plenty of nutritious food to compensate for the energy you burn during exercise. You will want to be sure you have a nice steady weight gain during your pregnancy. Your health-care provider will track your weight during your prenatal visits, and can help you determine whether you are gaining enough weight.

- Listen to your body, and take it easy when you need to. Remember that the purpose of exercise during pregnancy is to help keep you healthy, not to prepare you for the Olympics.

- If you experience any of the following symptoms, stop exercising and call your doctor for advice:
  ✓ Pain or difficulty walking
  ✓ Uterine contractions
  ✓ Vaginal bleeding or fluid loss
  ✓ Dizziness, faintness, or shortness of breath
  ✓ Rapid heart rate at rest
  ✓ A lack of movement in the baby

103 Weight Loss After Pregnancy: Self-Care Can Help You Balance the Demands of Parenting

A healthy weight gain supports a healthy pregnancy and a healthy baby. But once the baby is born, most women are eager to regain their pre-pregnancy figures. Following the birth of a baby, most women lose weight fairly quickly for the first three months. Weight loss then slows to about 1 or 2 pounds per month, until normal weight is achieved by about six months after the baby's birth.

Not every woman follows this pattern, however. Many women find that they are still carrying extra weight for a year or more after delivering their babies. Losing weight may be more challenging for you if you tend to gain weight easily, if you gained more than an average amount of weight during your pregnancy, or if you are still carrying extra weight six months or more after the birth of your baby. Following are some things to remember as you design a weight-control plan to take off those extra pounds.

Help your body heal during the first few months after your baby's birth.

The early postpartum period is not the time to rush into a demanding exercise program or a restrictive diet. During these early months, get plenty of rest, napping as much as possible. Get back into exercise slowly, following your doctor's recommendations for resuming activity, and eat as healthfully as possible. Be sure to drink plenty of water, especially if you are breastfeeding your baby.

Establish an exercise routine.

Regular physical activity should be the cornerstone of your weight control program. Exercise will help tone muscles, reduce fatigue, improve mood, and keep you healthy in many other ways. It will also burn some calories and enhance your weight loss efforts. You are most likely to stick to your exercise program if you make a plan for daily activity.

If you are new to exercise, start slowly and build gradually. What kind of activity can you fit into your new life? Walking is often the most accessible form of exercise, with or without baby in tow.

Breastfeeding moms can lose weight, too.

Some women who are breastfeeding worry that diet, exercise, and weight loss may compromise their milk supply, and the health of their babies. But research shows that as long as weight is lost slowly, and women are consuming a well-balanced diet, milk supply does not suffer. Similarly, exercise should be moderate, and balanced with adequate rest. Nurse your baby before exercising, so breasts will be more comfortable during exercise, and wear a supportive bra.

Build support for parenting and for your weight loss program.

Parenting is a 24-hour-a-day job. You can't do it alone. Get your partner, family, and friends to pitch in, if they can help. Or you may wish to join other new moms in a postpartum exercise class, if one is available in your area.

Reduce fatigue and stress.

Fatigue and stress are the most common reasons people go off their diets, or drop out of their exercise programs. They are also two of the things new parents all seem to have in common! Do everything you can to get enough rest and to reduce stress. Lower your expectations of what you can accomplish in a day. Enjoy your time with your baby as much as possible.

Eat sensibly, and avoid restrictive diets.

The best way to lose weight is to eat less and exercise more. The best way to eat less is to reduce the amount of empty calorie "junk" food in your diet. Try for a well-balanced diet that includes protein foods and carbohydrates at each meal, and eat plenty of fruits and vegetables.

Diets that restrict certain food groups often create cravings for those forbidden foods. Food restriction can also create feelings of stress and depression, which in turn may trigger overeating. You will be more successful in your weight loss efforts if you work with your body, and cultivate good eating habits that will be with you the rest of your life.

Remember that self-care is family-care.

Remember that you are a role model for your children. Boys and girls need to see a mom who models a healthful lifestyle that includes a good diet and regular physical activity. By making time to take care of yourself you will not only be a happier person, but you'll have more energy for the demands of your family, and you will inspire your children to be healthy as well.

Work and Family: Life in the Balance

For many people, juggling the multiple responsibilities of work and family life is a major source of stress. There just never seems to be enough time to get it all done. To make matters worse, we sacrifice sleep, relaxation and recreation to get our work done. What's wrong with this picture?

Trying to slow the pace of a lifestyle that feels out of control is no simple matter. When life starts to feel overwhelming, it pays to take some time to rethink your priorities, evaluate how you are using your time and be sure that at least the most important things are getting done. Some of the situations we find ourselves in may take a great deal of time and energy to sort out and simplify. Other times a few simple changes can at least give us room to take a few deep breaths, smell the flowers and slow down enough to enjoy the precious moments that make up a lifetime.

Your number-one priority is your health.

We take our health for granted, and forget that daily habits can enhance or erode our good health over the years. When there is too much to do in too little time, it is especially important to get enough sleep, eat well and exercise daily. And yet, during busy times, we tend to neglect our health. Remind yourself that to accomplish what needs to get done at work and at home, you must keep yourself in tip-top shape. You will make better decisions at work and at home, and have more energy for the people who are most important in your life.

Review your goals and priorities.

Your life has many important parts, including health, family, work, spiritual growth and recreation. Achieving balance means including activities that help you reach the most important goals in all parts of your life. Because work goals tend to be well defined for most people, it is easy to let these goals take priority over family goals and self-care.

You need to be your own boss when it comes to family goals. Schedule activities that will help you achieve these goals, and remember that these activities are just as important as your work activities. You may want to schedule family outings, family time for projects at home, and time with your spouse or partner.

Set realistic expectations.

Are your goals realistic? Can you fit everything in? If you are like most people, then probably not. Which goals and activities are the most important? Focus on making time for these.

Are some of your expectations causing you stress because they are unachievable in your present situation? Can you change the situation? If not, you may need to adjust your expectations to bring them closer to reality. What is a "good worker"? What is a "good parent"? What is a "good job"? What can you change to make your life simpler and less stressful? Get people to help you with what needs to get done.

Live your life.

Sometimes feelings of stress come from our own busy thoughts, thoughts that keep us so preoccupied that, when we are doing enjoyable things, we are not even there. Practice bringing mindful awareness to the present moment. Pay attention to what you are doing and the people you are with. Mindfulness helps reduce feelings of stress and slows busy, unproductive thoughts. Mindfulness also helps you enjoy special moments and think more clearly. This is your life, so enjoy it as much as possible! Laugh, have fun, and count your blessings.

Develop helpful routines and rituals.

Routines relieve stress, and rituals give life meaning. Routines reduce the need to make decisions when your mind is overcrowded. Autopilot can be great when it comes to everyone chipping in to clean up after dinner, planning meals, or getting out the door in the morning.

Pleasant routines can take on the quality of a ritual. After-dinner family activities, bedtime stories, and Saturday afternoon family hikes bring families together. Children especially need predictability and consistency, so our busy lives don't spill over and create hurried children.

Exercise Benefits for Midlife Women

Exercise does wonderful things for people of every age. Many exercise benefits are especially helpful to women as they navigate the transitions typical of midlife journeys— transitions that involve changing hormone levels, changing bodies, and changing lifestyles. Following are some of the most important exercise benefits for midlife women.

Exercise Helps Prevent Midlife Weight Gain

Many women (and men) notice a slow but steady weight gain during their midlife years. While some experts believe this weight gain may be caused in part by hormonal changes, others argue it is most likely due to a decreasing amount of muscle tissue, which in turn causes a decline in metabolic rate. Metabolic rate refers to the number of calories you burn each day. The more muscle you have, the more calories you burn.

Why do we lose muscle tissue over the years? While some of this loss is part of the aging process, more may be attributed to inactivity. Remember the "use it or lose it" rule of human physiology? Studies show that women who stay active throughout midlife have similar amounts of muscle tissue, similar metabolic rates and little midlife weight gain when compared to younger women. In other words, if you keep using those muscles, you will hold on to more of your muscle tissue as you age.

What if weight gain has already occurred? Whether you wish to prevent or reverse midlife weight gain, the answer is that old familiar refrain: exercise regularly and eat a healthful diet.

Exercise Improves Sleep and Lifts Fatigue

Many midlife women complain of trouble sleeping and daytime fatigue. While exercise may not prevent night sweats and hot flashes, it can improve sleep quality and daytime energy levels.

Exercise Helps Prevent and Treat Depression

Depression is no more common during midlife than at any other time of life. Women seek treatment for depression twice as often as men. Many symptoms of depression, such as muscle and joint pains, irritability, fatigue, changes in appetite and changes in sleeping habits, may be related to sleep disturbances. Midlife mood changes may also be related to changes in brain chemistry that occur with aging. Depression sometimes develops in response to loss, for example the death or illness of close friends and family members. In some cases, midlife depression is related to changing self-concept and life roles, as in the "empty nest" syndrome when women miss mothering their children who have grown up and left home. Whatever the cause, exercise combined with appropriate therapy helps relieve depression and its symptoms.

Exercise Boosts Self-Confidence

Exercise helps you look and feel your best at any age. Many midlife women get a tremendous boost in self-confidence after starting an exercise program, and they feel stronger in body, mind and spirit.

Exercise Slows Bone Loss

A woman's bone density begins to decline even before her midlife years, and this loss accelerates after menopause. All forms of exercise offer some protection against bone loss. Activities such as walking, jogging and strength training, which apply stress to the bones, help the most.

Women at high risk for osteoporosis may need more than exercise to keep their bones strong into old age, and should talk to their health-care providers about treatment and lifestyle options that may help to slow bone loss.

Exercise Helps Prevent Chronic Health Problems

Many health concerns become more of a reality in midlife. Fortunately, regular physical activity helps to prevent or delay the onset of a number of common chronic health conditions, including high blood pressure, Type 2 diabetes and artery disease. (Artery disease is the leading cause of heart disease and stroke.)

What Type of Exercise Program is Best?

An exercise program you can stick to is the best. If you are new to exercise, or making big changes in your program, check in with your doctor. You may also wish to work with a personal trainer to be sure your exercise program addresses your particular health concerns, fitness goals and lifestyle. If possible, try to exercise aerobically at least four days a week, and to perform strength-training exercises (to build muscle) at least two days a week. Stretch after your workouts to maintain flexibility. Most important, find activities you enjoy and have fun!

106 Does Menopause = Weight Gain?

As people grow older, they tend to lose muscle and bone mass, and gain fat. Because menopause coincides with these age-related changes for most women, it is tempting to blame all physical changes on "the change." Researchers believe, however, that lifestyle factors, in particular, diet and physical activity, have a stronger influence than estrogen levels on body weight and body composition. Studies show that women who remain active throughout the menopausal years have less likelihood of weight gain than their sedentary sisters. Following are some of the factors that help to explain the weight gain that is commonly attributed to menopause.

Accumulating Birthdays

People in their thirties begin losing around two or three pounds of muscle per decade. Over time, this results in a smaller amount of metabolically active tissue, and thus a significant drop in resting metabolic rate (the number of calories burned at rest). A lower metabolic rate means that you will gain weight unless you also decrease your calorie intake (how much you eat).

Fortunately, strength training can delay and reduce this loss of active muscle tissue. Thus, regular strength training helps prevent a decline in metabolic rate. It also helps keep muscles, joints, and bones strong and healthy.

Physical Activity

Physical activity burns calories. Physical activity includes not only exercise that you do to improve your fitness, but also daily activities like walking, chasing your kids around, housework, yard work and gardening. Many people gradually do less physical activity as the years go by. These changes mean fewer calories are burned. Even small changes in physical activity levels may be partly responsible for midlife weight gain, especially when combined with age-related decreases in metabolic rate.

Eating Habits

Eating habits may also change over time, and once again, small changes can accumulate into significant weight gain. Busy families may consume more fast food, women whose children have grown may have trouble reducing the amount of food they prepare, and large portion sizes in restaurants and at home encourage overeating at every age.

Ironically, years of low-calorie dieting can lead to midlife weight gain. Restrictive dieting can accelerate loss of muscle tissue and bone mass, which in turn lowers metabolic rate. Many dieters experience "rebound" weight gain as their bodies prepare for another round of starvation tactics. The best way to lose weight is by increasing physical activity and adopting healthful eating habits that lead to slow, but permanent fat loss.

Many midlife adults have been pleased to hear that alcohol may help reduce heart disease risk, and have added alcoholic beverages to their daily menu. Unfortunately, alcoholic beverages are high in calories, and excess alcohol calories seem to be more likely to be deposited around the middle.

Stress

People in midlife have no monopoly on stress. Each age group experiences various forms of stress that require energy and adaptation. Midlife stress wears many faces, and varies from person to person. Coping effectively with stress is important at any age. Chronic, uncontrollable stress is associated with many health problems such as high blood pressure, digestive disorders, depression, and anxiety. It also feels bad! Regular physical activity can help reduce feelings of stress and boost energy.

For some women, menopausal symptoms such as hot flashes, night sweats, and fatigue take a heavy toll on emotional wellbeing. Negative mood and fatigue are hard to live with, and interfere with plans to exercise and eat well. Women who find that menopausal symptoms are interfering with their lives should talk to their health-care providers, and discuss lifestyle and medical options for reducing the negative impact of these symptoms.

Hormones

While researchers studying menopausal weight gain do not place all of the blame on hormonal changes, they do acknowledge that changing hormone levels may play a role. We know that lower estrogen levels lead to an acceleration in the loss of bone density, and may cause other body composition changes as well. Many women do report gaining more fat in the abdominal region after menopause.

Preventing Weight Gain

The good news is that an active lifestyle, accompanied by healthful eating habits, can minimize midlife weight gain and changes in body composition. Be sure your exercise program is safe for you (check in with your health-care provider) and includes both aerobic and strength training exercise for maximum benefits.

107 Healthy Aging: Exercise and Good Nutrition Promote Health and Quality of Life

Scientists have yet to discover a true fountain of youth, but regular exercise and a healthful diet provide the best shot for staying as healthy as possible as we age. That's because some of the physical decline associated with the aging process is accelerated by a sedentary lifestyle and poor nutrition.

Exercise Benefits

Regular physical activity slows physical decline in many important ways. Both endurance exercise and strength training improve stamina, blood sugar regulation, resting blood pressure, artery health, and body composition. Strength training improves muscle size and strength, and prevents the frailty that can lead to falls and broken bones. While metabolic rate declines with age, exercise burns calories, which allows you to eat more food and thus get more nutrients from your diet.

Nutrition Needs Change With Age

Some things improve with age; unfortunately, the function of the digestive system is not one of them. Nutrient absorption tends to decline with age. In addition, most older adults need fewer calories than they did in early adulthood. Even with exercise, people experience some loss of muscle tissue and some reduction in metabolic rate. So the challenge for older adults is to get more nutrients with fewer calories and declining digestive function. Nutrient needs that change over time include the following:

- Vitamin D: Vitamin D is an important hormone that keeps people healthy in many ways, including maintenance of strong bones. While people can make vitamin D given enough sun exposure, the body becomes less efficient at doing this with age. Add sunscreen, cold weather, northern latitudes, and D production drops precipitously. Cow's milk and soy beverages are fortified with vitamin D, as are some breakfast cereals, types of orange juice, and yogurts. Adults over 70 should consume 1000 IUs of vitamin D per day. (Many experts now recommend this level for those over 50, too.)

- Vitamin B12: Absorption of this vitamin from food decreases in up to one third of older adults with a decrease in stomach acidity. B12 from supplements and fortified foods is more readily absorbed.

- Calcium: Calcium requirements increase from 1,000 to 1,200 mg at age 50, since absorption declines and loss of bone mineral accelerates, especially for women. Calcium should be consumed throughout the day, rather than taking one supplement once a day. Too much calcium can contribute to kidney stones and other health problems, so stay close to the requirement. A serving of dairy or calcium fortified foods gives you roughly 300 mg, and most people get at least 300 mg from the rest of their diet.

- Sodium: Sodium needs actually decline over time, as does the need for chloride. Older adults are more likely to experience high blood pressure with mineral imbalance (too much sodium and chloride, too little calcium, potassium, and magnesium). Salty foods are ubiquitous in the diet, and it takes real awareness and effort to decrease sodium intake.

Meals and snacks that consist primarily of things your ancestors would recognize as food provide the best nutrition: fruits, vegetables, whole grains, and lean protein sources. Strive for five to nine servings of fruits and vegetables each day. Plant foods provide many helpful vitamins, minerals, and fiber. The minerals in vegetables help to promote a more healthful acid-base balance in the body that prevents calcium being drawn from the bones. A multi vitamin and mineral supplement that provides the daily requirements for vitamins and minerals is good insurance. Choose one low in iron unless you have been told by your health-care provider to increase your iron intake.

Never Say Diet

Restrictive diets cause a loss of bone and muscle tissue that is difficult for older adults to regain. Such loss can accelerate the onset of osteoporosis and a progression into the frailty associated with old age. Restrictive diets rarely lead to successful, long-term weight control, since weight is regained (mostly as fat) once the diet is ended. To lose fat, increase your activity level and reduce food intake slightly by eating less of those foods you know you can do without (chips, desserts, etc.). Strength training will help prevent muscle and bone loss. Fat that is lost very slowly is more likely to stay off, and result in health benefits. An increase in activity will also improve health, even without any apparent change in weight.

Eat and Drink Like an Athlete

After exercise, enzymes responsible for muscle repair gear up for building muscle. Athletes often consume a protein and carbohydrate snack, beverage, or meal within an hour of physical activity to maximize the anabolic effects of exercise. And don't forget fluids. Thirst becomes a less reliable indicator of hydration with age. Try to consume at least four glasses of water a day, more with exercise.

You're Never Too Old to Exercise

Compare the effects of aging with those of exercise. With aging, you experience declines in muscle and joint strength, cardiovascular health and coordination. You lose muscle mass and gain fat. Chronic health problems, such as high blood pressure and diabetes, become more prevalent.

Enough of that. Let's talk about something more uplifting: exercise! Much of the decline in physical health and ability attributed to aging is accelerated by inactivity. While nothing can turn back the clock or make you live forever, a well-rounded exercise program can slow and even reverse many factors associated with the aging process.

Cardiovascular Health

Endurance exercise (also called aerobic exercise) and strength training improve cardiovascular health and help control several disorders that increase your risk of heart attack and stroke. Aerobic exercise refers to activities such as brisk walking or swimming that raise your metabolic rate for at least 10 minutes. These activities "stress" the muscles, bones and joints (the physiological systems that produce movement), the heart, blood vessels and lungs, and the other systems responsible for oxygen delivery and energy production. These systems respond to the stress of exercise by becoming stronger and healthier. Strength training refers to exercise that requires your muscles to exert a force against some form of resistance, such as weights, elastic tubing, water or the weight of your body, as in pushups.

With endurance and strength exercise, people with high blood pressure often see some reduction in both systolic and diastolic blood pressure. Blood sugar regulation improves, thus decreasing risk for type 2 diabetes or improving blood sugar control for people already diagnosed with diabetes. Exercise helps increase HDL cholesterol (the "good" kind) in the bloodstream, and helps lower blood triglycerides. Blood becomes less likely to form the kinds of clots that lead to heart attack or stroke inside the blood vessels. Regular exercise also burns calories and helps reduce excess body fat, especially when combined with a nutritious, low-fat diet. Regular exercise helps reduce the amount of fat stored inside the abdominal area. Excess fat in this location increases risk for diabetes, high blood pressure and heart disease.

Muscle and Joint Strength

People used to think that you can't teach old muscles new exercise tricks. Not so! It is now known that old muscles do respond to strength training by becoming larger and stronger.

The trick is to work fairly hard but not so hard as to cause an injury, such as a pulled muscle. A class or personal trainer may be helpful for beginners. Performing strength-training exercises two to three times a week for 20 to 30 minutes yields terrific results. Muscles and joints become stronger, daily activities feel easier, and balance improves, helping to prevent falls that can lead to broken bones.

What about flexibility? Many people find that their flexibility improves a little when they begin to exercise. Add 5 or 10 minutes of stretching exercises at the end of your exercise session for even more improvement.

Exercise as Physical Therapy

Exercise is often prescribed for orthopedic problems, such as rotator cuff injury, back aches and so forth. Many of the health problems that become more common with age—such as arthritis, insomnia, and diabetes—respond favorably to exercise. Be sure to include any therapeutic exercises you should be doing in your exercise program.

Mental Well-Being

Much research supports the connection between regular physical activity and psychological well being. Exercise helps prevent and treat depression. People who exercise regularly report feeling stronger, more energetic and more capable. Exercise helps relieve stress and improve quality of life. It has been said that while exercise may or may not add years to your life, it will certainly add life to your years.

You're Never Too Old

Unless you have a health problem that could be made worse by exercise (check with your doctor before starting an exercise program), you are never too old to start exercising. Begin slowly, build gradually and seek guidance from your doctor, exercise instructor, or personal trainer.

Seasonal Advice

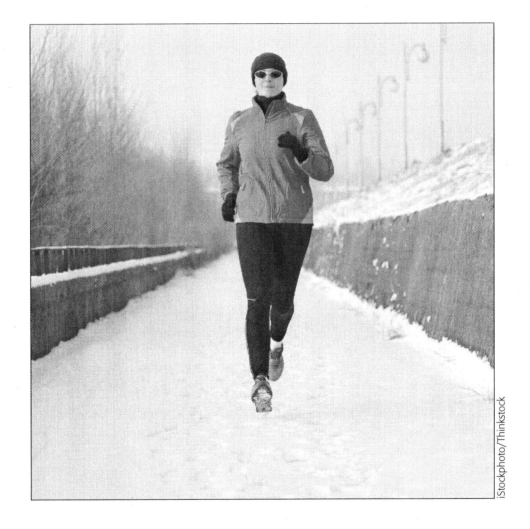

iStockphoto/Thinkstock

Chapter 9

Beat the Heat

When you're hot, you're hot, and prudent exercisers take the summer weather into account when setting up their exercise programs. Hot weather provides two challenges: avoiding dehydration and preventing dangerous elevations in internal temperature.

When you exercise, your muscles generate heat. Your circulatory system helps get rid of this excess heat by sending blood to the surface to release heat into the environment. People with fair skin will notice skin redness during and following exercise, especially in the face. That's a result of increased blood flow to the skin (unless it's a sunburn). The effectiveness of this method of heat release decreases as air temperature rises. Exercising with little or no air current also reduces the release of heat.

Heat may also be lost through the evaporation of sweat. Sweating is very effective when the air is dry, especially if there is a breeze. Hot, humid weather provides the biggest challenge to our cooling systems because heat is least effectively released to the environment.

Your risk of dehydration increases when you exercise in the heat. Dehydration is dangerous because it causes a decrease in blood volume. A lower blood volume means less circulation to the skin and possibly dangerous elevations in internal temperature.

There are many ways to beat the heat. Hot weather need not become an excuse to take a summer vacation from your exercise program. Following are a few suggestions for preventing heat stress and adapting your program to the demands of summer fun.

Drink plenty of fluids to prevent dehydration.

Exactly how much fluid you need to drink depends on your size, how much fluid your stomach can handle, your sweating rate, and environmental conditions. Nutritionists generally recommend 2 to 3 cups of water two hours before exercising in hot weather, then another 1 to 2 cups 15 minutes before your workout, depending upon how much you can tolerate without developing cramps. During your workout, continue to drink about 1 cup every 15 to 20 minutes. Cool drinks (40 to 50 degrees) are absorbed more quickly than lukewarm drinks.

Beware of early signs of dehydration.

Two good indicators of hydration are your body weight and urine output. Any weight lost during a workout is due to fluid loss. Weigh yourself before and after exercise, and drink the difference, about 2 cups for every pound. Monitor the volume and color of your urine. A pale color indicates normal water balance.

Recognize symptoms of heat illness.

Thirst, tiredness, disorientation, and visual disturbances can all point to heat illness. Stop exercising, drink something and find a cool place to rest. More drastic symptoms of heat exhaustion include a rapid, weak pulse, headaches, dizziness, and general weakness, and may require medical attention.

Consider environmental factors.

When deciding whether you should exercise outdoors, take all environmental factors into account, including temperature, humidity, the intensity of the sun, and how much the air is moving. Temperature alone does not tell the whole story. Heat stroke deaths have occurred during exercise in temperatures below 75 degrees Fahrenheit when the relative humidity was very high.

If heat is a problem, be creative. An air-conditioned fitness center is one answer. But getting outdoors is fun, too. Find a shadier walking route, go out early or late in the day, or exercise in the water.

Take into account your personal heat tolerance.

Several factors affect heat tolerance, including body composition, fitness level, and exposure.

Body Composition

Fat acts as insulation and slows heat loss to the environment, reducing heat tolerance. Larger people also expend more energy when performing a given amount of weight-bearing exercise, such as walking or aerobics. They, therefore, generate more muscle heat during such activities.

Fitness Level

If you are new to exercise, it may take you longer to get used to exercising in the heat. Take your time. Exercise will gradually get easier as you get in shape.

Exposure

People become acclimatized to warmer weather after exercising in it for about two weeks. The circulatory system becomes better able to handle the increased demands of heat release, and you begin sweating earlier and more heavily.

Recognize your own heat tolerance. Monitor your heart rate and stay within your target zone. You will find your heart rate rises faster than usual in the heat. The ability to exercise safely in the heat varies considerably from person to person. It is important to know your own limits so that summer exercise is safe and fun.

110 Travel Plans? Don't Forget to Include Exercise

We rely on the force of habit to support our healthful lifestyles. Our routine gets us to the fitness center, helps us choose nutritious meals, and cope effectively with stress. Anything that disrupts our routine, such as travel, vacations, holidays, and even visitors, can send that lifestyle into a tailspin. While a week or two away from exercise probably does little harm, it's discouraging to feel that hard-earned improvements are being reversed. When travel plans are on the horizon, why not plan to take advantage of the change in routine to reaffirm your commitment to a healthful lifestyle?

Plan ahead.

It's not enough to tell yourself, "I'll try not to overeat" or "I will try to walk every day." Most people need more concrete guidelines. Think about where you will be. How will you cope with too much food? How, when and where will you exercise? Write up a specific plan. Some people find it motivational to share this plan with an instructor, trainer or partner.

Record your progress while you're on the road.

Once you have a plan, design a simple form or use a calendar to record your workouts and other behaviors (food intake, for example, if that's a concern). Keep your log in a convenient place where you'll see it every day.

Anticipate and plan for potential difficulties.

As you make travel plans, hope for the best but be prepared for problems that inevitably arise. For example, if your plan is a daily walk outdoors, what will you do when it rains? Take along a raincoat or umbrella, or be prepared to use the exercise machines at the hotel. Having anticipated problems, you will be less likely to throw in the towel when challenges arise.

Get support from family, friends, and coworkers.

Let your family, friends or those you are traveling with know about the importance of your exercise program. Business travelers may be able to recruit coworkers for an early morning walk or workout to plan the day. Vacationers can try to get family and friends involved as exercise partners or as a support system to provide a temporary release from childcare or other duties.

Try to find environments that support a healthful lifestyle.

When making vacation plans, consider options that offer opportunities for enjoyable physical activities. Most cruises and resorts provide exercise facilities and classes. Campers can select locations with beautiful hiking or biking trails. Headed to the coast? What's better than a walk along the beach? If children will be along, figure out a way to be active as a family; take along bikes, strollers, child carriers, or whatever is needed for mobility. Business travelers may be able to select a hotel that offers at least an exercise machine or two.

Do all you can to stay healthy.

Catching a cold can really upset an exercise program, not to mention make you feel lousy. Somehow it's easier to get sick while traveling. Perhaps jet lag, sleep loss, dehydration and exposure to new germs impose excess stress on the immune system. Do what you can to avoid getting sick. Wash your hands frequently, drink plenty of water, get enough sleep, avoid drinking too much alcohol, and take your vitamins.

Use exercise to manage the stress of traveling.

Travel means change, and change, even positive change, is a form of stress that requires some adjustment. Travel presents new situations that require problem-solving ranging in difficulty from simple, like ordering from a new menu, to complex, like losing your wallet. Everyone knows that physical activity is one of the most effective stress-management techniques around. When things do not go exactly as they should, you may be tempted to skip your workout because you're feeling stressed. If this happens, remind yourself that exercise will help relieve those feelings of stress and improve your problem-solving ability so you can better cope with the inevitable challenges and opportunities of travel.

111 Positive Emotions: An Antidote to Holiday Stress

The holiday season is fast approaching, and with it the joy and hope that are a meaningful part of holiday traditions. But for many of us, the holidays also bring stress: too much to do in too little time, loneliness, or disappointment that life is not as it should be. Sometimes the joy and wonder get overlooked because we are hurried or distracted.

Too much stress reduces quality of life, and puts a damper on holiday spirits. It can also contribute to health problems. Research has found that negative emotions, such as fear, anger, and sadness, are associated with poorer immune function, and increased risk of illness. Stress contributes to high blood pressure, digestive disorders, and muscle tension, as the body continually tenses for action, ready to fight or flee. Many people attempt to reduce feelings of stress in ways that further worsen health: eating and drinking too much, or smoking.

You can reduce feelings of stress by making time for self-care, creating opportunities to focus on the positive things in life, and taking time to do things you enjoy. Positive emotions, such as love, joy, and contentment counteract the negative effects of stress. They enhance immune function and improve your ability to cope with challenging situations. They also nourish your holiday spirit!

Make time for self-care.

Self-care provides essential energy to recharge your spirit. It's hard to feel pleasure when you are run down and exhausted. Maybe you can't squeeze in a day at the spa, but make time for a hot bath or a delicious healthy meal with family or friends.

Stick to your exercise program as much as possible. Physical activity relieves stress and reduces feelings of anger and irritability that can arise with overload. Exercise helps you feel energized in a calm and focused way, so you can be productive without feeling so stressed about it. Exercise also contributes to good health, strengthening the immune system and counteracting stress-related illnesses such as high blood pressure and heart disease. And since good food abounds during the holidays, you may need to burn extra calories to prevent winter weight gain.

No time for your regular workout schedule? Then try for shorter sessions, but at least do something. If you are in good shape, increase exercise intensity to compensate for a shorter exercise duration. Make opportunities for physical activity over the holidays: get everyone out for a walk, take the children sledding, or go dancing.

Encourage friends and family to make self-care a priority. Need a gift idea? How about self-care gift certificates: for a massage, hot tub, or personal-training sessions.

Use mindful awareness to see the positive.

Have you ever done something "fun," but been so preoccupied you didn't enjoy it? In order to experience positive emotions you need to be in a positive place, but you also have to be in the moment, so you are able to appreciate what's going on. Sometimes when people are busy this is hard to do.

You can practice mindful awareness in simple ways. Eat slowly and savor a piece of fruit or a meal. Breathe deeply and tune in to the way your body is feeling. Watch the birds at the bird feeder or the squirrels on the lawn, and try not to think of anything else for five minutes. If you are like most people, your mind may try to race away into the past or the future. Don't be surprised, and don't get frustrated. Simply bring your awareness back to the present.

You can observe your emotions in this same way throughout the day. Sometimes you can choose to not dwell in negative emotions such as anger or sadness, especially if it's just something small (or even just your thoughts) setting these emotions off. Take a minute to focus instead on the things you are grateful for and on the people you love, and the things that give your life meaning.

Mindful awareness can help you slow down and appreciate the richness of life. Instead of just trying to "survive" or "make it through" the holidays, why not try to create a meaningful holiday season for yourself and those you love? Do less and enjoy more.

Make time for pleasure.

Pleasurable experiences reduce stress and feel good! Enjoy your daily pleasures, such as a delicious cup of tea, a good book by the fire, a delicious meal. Laughter is especially therapeutic—watch a funny movie and read the comics. Feeling good will reduce holiday stress and get you off on the right foot in the New Year.

Energize Your Holiday Spirit

It happens every year: the holiday season arrives, with its hustle, bustle, and extra demands on your time, energy, and good humor. Following are a few suggestions for mobilizing the energy and enthusiasm it takes to create and sustain that holiday spirit.

Energize with exercise.

Instead of reaching for caffeine, get out for a walk or an exercise class. It's easy to drink too much caffeine when you're on holiday overload, when summoning the energy to get through the day feels like squeezing water from a stone. While too much caffeine makes you tired and wired, a good workout helps you feel physically relaxed but mentally alert. It relieves feelings of tension and stress, and helps you concentrate. And, unlike caffeine, it enhances sleep quality and offers wonderful health benefits.

For some people, holidays bring unpleasant reminders of passing time, and especially sadness that certain loved ones are no longer with us. Exercise helps reduce feelings of depression. Activities that get you out of the house and break the cycle of depressing thoughts are especially helpful.

Get your "40 winks."

If fatigue is a problem, sleep may be the answer. When there aren't enough hours in the day, you may be tempted to steal some from the night. But even a few short nights can dampen your energy and enthusiasm, especially when demands on your time require you to perform in high gear all day long. Adequate quality sleep restores your energy and optimism.

Diet: Balance indulgence with moderation.

Delicious treats abound during the holiday season. Make conscious choices regarding indulgences, and eat to celebrate. Certain foods add life and meaning to the holidays—these you cannot go without. Others are kind of just there. Avoid snacking on junk you don't really want. You will enjoy the really special treats more if your diet has been relatively well-balanced overall. Your exercise program will help you accommodate a few extra calories. A balanced diet helps you avoid the fatigue and irritability associated with low blood-sugar levels and hunger, and that overstuffed, sleepy feeling of eating too much.

Be alert to early signs of stress.

Sometimes, our bodies tell us we're under stress before we are willing to acknowledge it. We bite our nails, get headaches, drink too much or misplace things more than usual. Nipping excess stress in the bud is more effective than trying to cope with a field gone to seed. Change the things you can change. Figure out why you are feeling stressed, and address the situation. Too busy? Find ways to do less and enjoy more. If loneliness is the source of stress, look for opportunities to volunteer to help those less fortunate. If you can't change the source of stress, try changing your attitude. Get the most out of the things you can't change.

Prioritize: Make time for the things that are most important.

Where will the time come from? From the time you don't lose by getting sick. Make taking care of yourself a priority. Getting sick can really deflate your holiday spirit. Get enough rest, eat well, exercise and manage stress. In addition, see if you can get rid of or postpone any projects. If something simply won't get done, decide what that something should be.

For most people, special activities are part of the holiday tradition. Make time for these. Getting together with family and friends reinforces those vital connections that enhance the quality of life and provide buffers during times of stress. Do what you can to make gatherings quality time for yourself and those you care about. At parties, get help with preparation and cleanup; try potluck this year. Turn off the television. Play games. Spend quality time with the friends and family members you love the most. Look for the positive, and remember that the holiday season comes but once a year and will be over sooner than you think.

113 Holiday Indulgence: Guilt-Free Eating for the Holiday Season

Food and holidays go hand in hand. Special foods are part of the reason holidays are special. While the warm glow that holiday treats add to family and community togetherness is good for your health, weeks of overindulgence in delicious desserts is not.

Let's admit it: Traditional holiday fare is not known for being particularly low in fat, sugar or salt, or high in fiber or essential nutrients.

Holidays should be a time of celebration, but for some, the holiday season becomes a battleground where vigilant self-control is under constant siege from irresistible culinary temptation. Consider these suggestions for healthful and guilt-free holiday eating and enjoyment.

Eat for the right reasons.

During the holidays, we share good food with friends. Celebration of holiday rituals requires appropriate indulgence. Certain foods symbolize holiday meaning in many cultures and families. Enjoy! Join in the festivities and savor the delicious fare.

Beware, however, of using the holidays as an excuse for over-indulgence. Two or three potato latkes are enjoyable, but remember they are fried. You wouldn't miss a slice of your great aunt's pecan pie, but a thin slice is preferable to a fourth of the pie. Holiday fun includes more than eating.

Make conscious choices.

When you are surrounded by appealing treats, it can be difficult to figure out what you really want to eat. Realizing that one of each will be too many, go for a few of what you want the most. In other words, don't just walk into the room and start eating. If you really want the pumpkin cookies, it's better to have a few rather than munching on vegetables and dip, a turkey sandwich, and then finally getting to the cookies, which were all you really wanted in the first place.

Conscious choice also means having an awareness of your food selections during the day, and even the week. A late-afternoon party can be followed by a light dinner. If Friday and Saturday are heavy party days, accentuate the steamed vegetables and salads at meals early in the week. You will enjoy the treats more if they are special, not daily fare.

Exert control over what kinds and amounts of treats you wish to have around the house. Keep them out of view, and reserved for special occasions. Bake cookies, and then give most of them away. Be sure to have plenty of healthful snacks on hand. Often, you can choose between high- and low-fat alternatives. For example, choose hot mulled cider over eggnog. Or if eggnog is essential, choose low-fat eggnog over the high-fat variety.

Cultivate a repertoire of healthful treats.

Holiday treats can be good for you. Many wonderful cookbooks present delicious but healthful recipes. Start some new holiday traditions that offer health, as well as good taste. Remember, these treats must be treats; you must perceive these healthful foods as nourishing and delicious, not as poor second cousins to what you would rather have.

Take care of yourself to diminish the need for emotional eating.

Many people overeat during the holidays because they need to feed a hungry heart. Holidays bring stress and sorrow, as well as joy. Pamper yourself with a hot bath, a good book or a long walk with a best friend. Try to give yourself a realistic schedule. If you don't have time for everything, decide to do less and enjoy yourself more.

Get enough sleep.

It's easy to miss out on sleep during this season of parties, travel, visitors and too much to do. But adequate sleep is essential for good health and stress management. Here's another reason to get enough sleep: Studies have shown that people short on sleep eat more, almost as though trying to obtain the energy from food that was meant to come from adequate rest.

Keep exercising.

You need exercise during the holiday season more than ever to help manage holiday stress and to balance an increased energy intake.

Resolutions for a New Year: Fitness Success

A new year, a new calendar, a fresh new start. Anything is possible, and after the excesses of the holiday season many of us feel the urge to turn over a new leaf. But it takes more than a New Year's resolution to create successful, long-term changes in behavior. Your New Year's resolutions are most likely to become a new way of life if you spend some time thinking about how you will reach your resolution goals. Research has shown that people who take some time to make a concrete plan and anticipate possible difficulties are more likely to stick to their New Year's resolutions long after the January page on the calendar has been turned.

Make physical activity the foundation of your behavior change program.

Regular physical activity is an essential component of any weight loss program. Exercisers also have twice the success in trying to quit smoking as do their sedentary friends. Physical activity reduces feelings of stress, and increases feelings of energy and control. Regular physical activity has enormous fringe benefits including better health and greater vitality.

Make your health and well-being a priority.

Many people find they put their own needs on hold to take care of all the urgent matters that arise at work, at home, and in their communities. They take their health for granted, until it isn't there. Why wait to get sick to start taking care of yourself? Remember that an ounce of prevention is worth a pound of cure. By exercising and eating well now, you may save yourself hours (even years) of time in the future.

Change for the right reasons.

The right reasons are positive, and based on the belief that you deserve a little time each day to help keep yourself healthy. When you take a little time to nurture yourself, you will have more to give to the people and things you care about—your family, your work, and your community.

Wrong reasons focus on self-blame and guilt and lead to low self-esteem and negative feelings. They make you feel bad, and when you feel bad, you lose the motivation to exercise, or to follow through with other actions to improve your health.

Prepare for change.

Change is not always comfortable and easy. Adding physical activity to your life requires both time and energy.

Where will the time come from? How will you summon the energy? Make a concrete plan for fitting exercise into your life.

Then take a critical look at your plan. Is it realistic? People beginning the new year often overestimate their powers, and underestimate the time and energy required to stick to their resolutions. If your goals are too unrealistic (you probably won't lose 30 pounds in 30 days), you will quickly be disappointed. Set attainable goals. For example, many experts recommend that instead of a weight loss goal, make your goal the lifestyle change itself: enjoying daily physical activity, and eating less junk. If you are successful in achieving these daily goals, the weight loss will gradually follow.

You may wish to get some help as you prepare for change. Find out about opportunities for physical activity in your community and at work. Consider taking an exercise class, joining a fitness center, or working with a personal trainer. Ask a friend or family member with similar interests to join you and be your exercise partner. If you have health concerns, talk to your health-care provider before increasing your level of vigorous physical activity.

Anticipate difficulties.

Make plans to get back into your program when it is interrupted for illness, travel, weather, or the million other details that arise. Remember, it's not a question of whether you will have to skip an exercise session, but a question of what you will do when this happens. Avoid all or nothing thinking. Everyone misses a workout from time to time.

What are the reasons that have kept you from exercising in the past? How did you respond? Are there ways to keep these difficulties from arising? Or ways to exercise despite these challenges? Use your creative problem solving abilities to anticipate difficulties. If you stop exercising for some reason, how will you get back into your exercise routine as soon as possible?

Get moving!

If exercise is new to you, start slowly and build gradually. Record your workouts in an exercise log, and be proud of your progress. Enjoy the way exercise gives you energy and reduces stress. From time to time, consider what's working and what's not working with your exercise routine. Do everything you can to make regular physical activity a lifelong habit.

Working With Your Resolutions: Revamp and Revise for Maximum Effect

How about those New Year's resolutions? Are you making some progress toward your behavior change goals? Whether you have resolved to lose weight, exercise more, spend more time with your family, or get more recognition at work, setting goals and making plans are an important part of life, not just in January, but all year round.

Resolutions reflect our need for improvement in our lives. Resolutions help us feel like we have some control over our lives, and that we can make our lives better. For this reason, making resolutions helps us feel optimistic and reduces feelings of stress.

But sticking to those resolutions is another story. By the end of January, many people have thrown their resolutions out the window because they felt unable to achieve their expectations. Not achieving our goals produces stress, lowers self-esteem, and makes us feel frustrated, disappointed, and angry with ourselves.

This is no way to start a new year! If your resolutions are still something you would like to achieve but you are having difficulty making changes, take a moment to re-evaluate your resolutions. The following questions may help you revamp and revise your resolutions to achieve more success.

Is your resolution something you really want?

Your goal should be something really meaningful for you and something you really want to achieve. Spend some time thinking about your goals in life. What kind of resolution would help you get there?

Some people get mad at their resolutions because, in reality, the goal is not something they really want, but something they think they should want. For example, some people think they should lose weight because someone else, usually a significant other, has suggested this. But this suggestion may have felt more like criticism than a good idea, so the resolution carries too many negative overtones that create stress and reduce motivation.

Is your resolution stated in a positive way?

Resolutions that have a helpful, positive ring to them are most effective. "I will try to speak more kindly about others" is better than "I'll try not to gossip about other people so much." "I'll try to eat more healthful foods" creates a positive idea, while "I will not eat desserts" makes us feel deprived. As soon as we can't have something, we seem to just want it more!

Was your resolution feasible?

Grandiose resolutions sound great and make us feel good when we say them to ourselves. But if your resolution is too unrealistic, it won't be helpful because you won't stick to it. Be sure your resolution is something you can achieve.

If your goal no longer seems feasible, try toning it down a bit. Better to achieve a little progress with a modest but feasible goal than achieve nothing with an overly ambitious one. For example, if you resolved to exercise an hour every day, but just can't make the time, how about shooting for half an hour a day, or an hour three days a week?

Did you make a specific plan for achieving your goals?

You can only reach a goal if you have a good action plan, doable steps that help you move toward your goal. This is where goals most often fail. Without a concrete set of directions you are likely to get lost, or perhaps not even know how to get started.

If you need a better plan, make time to think about the best ways to reach your goal. You may wish to break your big goal into smaller, more achievable goals. Turn each goal into a series of specific steps. Make a list of activities that will move you toward your goal. Write them down. Then schedule these activities into your life.

Do you have a way to measure your progress?

Tracking your progress is very motivational. Keep a record of the behavior you are trying to change. For example, if you want to exercise more, keep an exercise log.

What have you learned from your attempts to stick to your resolution?

If you are still trying to stick to your New Year's resolution, what's working? What's not working? If you have tried to achieve this same or a similar goal in the past, what has been helpful? What factors have gotten in the way? Learn from these experiences, and adjust your goal and action plans accordingly.

Do you need more support?

Find or create a support group, or a group with the same goal as you. Ask your family for help. Get a friend to join you in your efforts. You may have more fun and be more successful as well!

Making Friends With Winter

For most healthy people, winter is no excuse to get cold feet about outdoor exercise. Staying indoors, and not getting enough fresh air, exercise, and exposure to natural light, can lead to seasonal depression, as well as general grumpiness. Our animal instincts say "hibernate." We tend to eat more and gain a few pounds. Regular exercise can help hoist us out of the winter blues and help us make friends with winter.

Embrace the change.

Instead of regarding winter as an unfortunate barrier, find something about it to like. If you regard winter weather as a curse to be endured, you make yourself winter's hostage, resentful of its icy grasp. A positive attitude helps people cope with the challenges of winter conditions.

Need motivation? Consider the results of one study that compared exercise energy expenditure for room temperature and cold environments. A given amount of exercise in the cold burned about 13 percent more calories.

Exercise caution.

Some health conditions are not compatible with cold, dry air. People with asthma may be better off enjoying winter through the windows as they swim indoors or workout on indoor exercise equipment. People with high blood pressure and heart disease should check with their doctors about exercising in the cold. While exercise may provide a healthy stress, the additional stress of a cold environment may produce system overload.

Early darkness and dangerous surfaces make some activities not worth the risk. Cycling after dark is 15 to 20 times more dangerous than daylight riding. Pedestrian injuries are also much more common at night. Stay away from traffic and icy spots. Head for the ski slopes or cross-country ski trails.

Dress for success.

Appropriate attire can help you exercise comfortably and safely. When dressing to go outdoors, consider the intensity of the upcoming activity. People new to cold weather exercise often overdress, get hot and sweaty, remove layers too late, and then get chilled. When you first go outside to exercise, you should feel slightly cool. You'll warm up after a few minutes. Open a zipper or take off a layer the minute you start to sweat.

Layers help you adapt your clothing to your needs. If you have one heavy coat over a t-shirt, modifications are limited. If, instead, you have a turtleneck, light sweatshirt, vest, and a windbreaker, you can fine-tune your attire for comfort.

If you are in the market for some new exercise clothes, consider thermal under layers made of fabrics that wick away perspiration from the skin. Perspiration is designed to cool you; wet clothes transfer heat from your body to the air. Your winter dressing goal is to stay dry and warm, but not hot. Another handy wardrobe addition is a jacket made of breathable material that keeps the wind and rain out, but allows perspiration to evaporate.

Don't let a lack of high-tech clothing keep you indoors, however. People have been enjoying winter sports for years, long before these fabrics came along. Use whatever you have and over time you can gradually modify your exercise wardrobe so that it works for you.

Prevent cold injury.

Your hands, toes, ears, and nose are most vulnerable to frostbite. In the cold, your body shuts down blood flow to the skin, where valuable heat is lost. Even though most of you feels warm, extremities can still suffer frostbite. Warning signs are numbness and a white appearance. Wear gloves or mittens, warm shoes and socks, and something over your ears to prevent frostbite in these areas. Your nose may need covering, as well, on very cold or windy days. Circulation to the head does not slow down in the cold; your brain must continue to function. Wear a hat to prevent heat loss from the head.

Warm up for the cold.

Warm up indoors by jogging in place, or walking up and down the stairs. Now you are ready to keep moving once you're outdoors. After your workout, cool down as you near the indoors, and stretch inside. Beware of sun damage, especially if it is snowy, and wear sunglasses and sunscreen. And don't forget that you still need extra fluids in the cold. Water is lost through perspiration and respiration as your lungs humidify the cold, dry air.

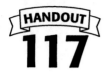

Prevent Winter Weight Gain

Many people gain weight during the winter months. Some joke that they are eating and sleeping more because they are getting ready to hibernate. But we do not get to crawl into a warm hiding place and sleep the fat away! So in our sedentary culture, where over half of all adults are already overweight, factors that accelerate weight gain are a real concern. Those extra pounds acquired over the winter may stay on year after year, eventually contributing to health problems such as obesity, diabetes, high blood pressure, and heart disease.

People tend to gain weight during the winter months for many different reasons. If you have a tendency to gain weight during the winter, it's important for you to figure out what factors contribute to this tendency, and then plan accordingly. Simple changes in behavior often have enormous health benefits. Following are some ideas for preventing winter weight gain. As you read, decide which would be helpful for you.

Make a holiday survival plan.

When you think about it, it is remarkable that some people do *not* gain weight during the holidays! Holidays can mean less time to exercise, more treats, and extra alcohol and stress that trigger overeating. You couldn't find a better recipe for weight gain. If your winter weight gain tends to come on during the holiday season, then consider making a holiday survival plan.

First, come up with a plan for staying active. Think about factors that have made exercise during the holiday season difficult in the past: loneliness, travel, busy-ness, lack of childcare, or whatever. Try to come up with some creative solutions, then schedule them into your calendar the same way you schedule parties, meetings, and family gatherings.

Second, think of ways to reduce holiday stress, if the holidays create excess stress for you. Exercise is the best stress reducer around, and stress reduction is one of the best reasons to stay active no matter what the season may be. Also important are getting enough sleep, focusing on your priorities, and eliminating low-priority activities if you are too busy. Make time for those activities that give the holidays meaning and provide pleasure and opportunities to be with people you enjoy.

Third, eat defensively. Include occasional small portions of holiday treats that you really love, but balance your intake by eating more prudently at other meals. Avoid munching and drinking just because "it's there." If you drink alcohol, keep consumption reasonable.

Make friends with winter.

Winter can cause a decline in physical activity level, as shorter days and inclement weather limit exercise options. If winter weather creates exercise barriers for you, take a closer look at those barriers and come up with some creative alternatives. If early darkness forces you off the streets, how about some indoor options? Check out fitness centers and community recreation programs in your area, and move your exercise program indoors.

Are you afraid of the cold? Buy some warmer clothes, and learn how to dress for cold weather. If you are lucky enough to have some snow, learn a winter sport. Cross-country skiing, ice-skating, and snowshoeing are terrific calorie-burners and are easy to learn.

Winter doldrums? Get into the light.

Many people experience mild to moderate winter depression. Severe winter depression, known as Seasonal Affective Disorder (SAD) is marked by depressed mood, sleeping more than usual, increased appetite, cravings for sweets and carbohydrates, and weight gain. If depression is a problem for you, talk to your health-care provider. Providers may recommend some form of light therapy, which relieves winter depression in many people.

Don't forget that exercise can be an effective treatment for mild to moderate depression. People who experience winter depression can try combining exercise and light therapy by exercising outdoors when time and weather permit.

More Advice

Barry Austin

If you are a fitness enthusiast, you may find it hard to understand why other people don't get it. Exercise has so many benefits, and makes you look and feel so good, why doesn't everyone get out and move it? You may especially wonder about family members, and your good friends. Is there any way to help them see the light?

Advice on Giving Advice

Don't. People generally dislike being given advice or told what to do, especially by family members and friends. Think about the last time someone tried to give you advice when you hadn't asked for any. Generally, we take these directives as criticism, and put up a wall of defense to preserve our self-esteem. We reject the advice, and sometimes the advice giver as well. Instead of launching into a lecture, take a moment to think about the behavior change process and how you can best encourage your friend to become more active.

Understanding Behavior Change

Behavior change begins in the brain. People must first see a good reason to change their comfortable habits. They weigh the pros and cons, and if the pros are strong enough, they decide to change.

What does this have to do with your friend? Dragging unwilling friends to the fitness center may not be productive in the long run. First, find out if they are really interested in becoming more active, and what types of activity would be the most fun for them.

Information helps people consider changing, but emotion is a stronger factor. People can forget or ignore information, but if the information touches something they care about, it is more likely to lead to change. If people see exercise as a way to have more self-confidence for a job search, or more energy to play with grandkids, they may experience more motivation to become more active.

The Decision to Change

What if your friend does not want to exercise? You can bug them a little bit, but don't overdo it. Do you have a short article on exercise benefits they might read? Would exercise help a health problem that concerns them? Would they tolerate small amounts of activity that does not feel too inconvenient (a walk at lunchtime)? If your suggestions do not take hold, let it go, and try again in a month or two. Your friend may continue to consider the nudge you have given, and come around later.

Focus on behavior, not weight loss.

If your friend is trying to lose weight, resist asking how much weight he or she has lost this week. Weight loss may occur very slowly. Instead, focus on the lifestyle behaviors your friend is trying to change, such as eating better and exercising regularly. Choose nutritious meals if you eat out together, and don't sabotage their efforts by giving them junk food. Take a walk or bike ride together.

Build self-efficacy.

Self-efficacy is psycho-jargon for a can-do attitude. People are more likely to stick to an exercise program if they believe they can. To increase self-efficacy, help your friend successfully complete small steps that demonstrate competence.

False praise doesn't work. Pointing out the facts does. "Look, you say you can't work exercise into your day, but this week we've walked after work three times!" Express sincere confidence in their abilities, and be supportive.

This sounds easy, but often we focus more on ourselves, wanting to show friends how fit we are, how much we know, how accomplished we are. Many friends are fairly competitive with each other. To build self-efficacy in others, you have to help them shine.

Suspend judgment, and be a friend.

If friends have had a bad day, and have not exercised as planned, be sympathetic rather than judgmental. After all, you are a friend, so show your understanding that we all have bad days. Invite them out for a nice walk to help manage stress! Your relationship is probably built on enjoying time together. Create ways to be together that involve some activity.

Ask your friend to help you.

Is there a way your friend could help you that would get them moving? Some people exert more effort to help another than to take care of themselves. Do you need more activity to strengthen your bones, manage stress, or lower your cholesterol? Get your friend to work out with you.

What if you are worried about your friend?

If you are really worried about your friend because of a health problem, physical or psychological, urge that friend to make an appointment with the doctor. Make the appointment, and go with your friend, if this is possible. Even the best of friends can't solve every problem; people must confront these themselves, and professional support is helpful.

119 Too Good to Be True? Protect Yourself From Health Fraud

People in North America spend billions of dollars each year on fraudulent products that deliver only empty promises, never living up to their advertising claims. Some of the most popular are devices and supplements to help you lose weight, tone up muscles, and boost metabolism. These products are a waste of money, and can even be harmful to your health.

Fraudulent products often masquerade as alternative medicine. But while some alternative approaches to healing have been studied and are supported by scientific studies, fraudulent products are pure advertising, with no evidence to support their safety or efficacy. Following are some ways to spot a health fraud.

Claims are too good to be true.

One product often promises to cure everything from obesity to arthritis to cancer, quickly and easily. The advertising literature for some of these products is many pages long, featuring a different health problem on each page. One product is promoted to cure them all. Words such as "miraculous," "dramatic," and "unbelievable" are used to describe the results. Claims of cure are often wildly extravagant.

Advertising encourages suspicion of the medical establishment.

People and groups promoting fraudulent products often claim the products are being suppressed by physicians and the pharmaceutical industry. They suggest that the medical establishment wants to keep you sick in order to make a profit. While we have all run into a difficult doctor from time to time, most medical professionals make a living by helping to heal the sick. Like all scientists, most doctors are suspicious of unproven treatments, and for good reason. Many of these treatments are not only ineffective, but harmful as well.

Products lack valid scientific support.

Scientists publish their research in scientific journals. Their work is closely reviewed by other scientists to be sure it is accurate and valid. Newspaper and magazine articles, television interviews, and infomercials do not count as valid scientific support. Neither do unpublished studies. Because these products are loosely regulated, outrageous advertising may continue for many months until a regulatory agency catches on, and calls a halt. At this point, the damage is done and the profits spent. So remember: it's just advertising.

Advertising relies heavily on testimonials of individuals who have used the product.

Some people may believe that the product has worked for them, but the improvement of a few individuals does not indicate that the product really works. Here's why.

A person using a product may experience improvement for many reasons. Many illnesses have periods of remission, or go away on their own; the user's symptoms may have subsided without the product. The power of belief, called the placebo effect, is very strong. People who believe they will feel better usually do, even if they are given an inactive sugar pill.

Many fraudulent products and therapies are administered by well-meaning but uneducated individuals. Consumers interpret and respond to this intention to help by wanting to reciprocate, and feel better. We may perceive improvements when none have actually occurred.

Improvement may occur for other reasons as well. People often use fraudulent products along with other therapies, or change other behaviors during the time they are using the product. Many weight loss products take advantage of this fact, and recommend that you follow a low-calorie diet while using the product. Which caused the weight loss, the product or the diet? Probably the diet.

Products are heavily advertised for a relatively short period of time, and then disappear.

Effective products can stand the test of time. Support for them grows as time goes by. Products that quickly appear and disappear are often someone's attempt to make some quick money. Products sometimes disappear quickly because a regulatory agency such as the Food and Drug Administration or the Federal Trade Commission has received complaints of health fraud for that product. Time to close up shop!

Health Advice for Frequent Flyers

People whose jobs in the global marketplace require frequent travel face many health challenges. Jet lag leads the list, as abrupt changes in the light-dark cycle disrupt our internal biological clocks, and leave us feeling foggy and disoriented. Noisy accommodations, restaurant dining, too much caffeine and alcohol, and frantic schedules compound jet lag fatigue. Add a little bad weather, travel delays, or a nasty cold ... are we having fun yet?

Cope with jet lag.

We live in a world whose natural cycles reflect the rhythm of day and night. Over evolutionary time, animals, including humans, have adapted to the 24-hour cycle of light and dark. All of our physical and mental functions are governed by this cycle, from bowel function and hormone production to mental alertness and reaction time.

While the light-dark cycle changes gradually with the seasons, it is only in very recent history that our bodies have had to adjust to sudden changes in this cycle. Some people seem to adapt to time zone changes more easily than others, but almost everyone experiences a feeling of being out of sync when traveling more than a time zone or two.

The best way to reset your internal clock is to get back into a daily schedule as soon as possible. Regular physical activity and exposure to daylight can also help your body recover more quickly from jet lag.

Schedule daily physical activity.

Frequent flyers need strategies for staying active when they are away from home. Exercise helps you cope with jet lag, strengthens your immune system, and makes you feel more energetic and focused, so that your work (and play!) time is productive.

Daily physical activity will only occur if you take control and schedule it into your day. Before leaving home, consider your exercise options, and plan them into your workday. Can you stay in a hotel with a fitness center? Are there interesting places to walk and sight see? Hike? Golf? If you are traveling to a new location, explore activity options with your local contacts. What will fit into your schedule?

What time of day is best? Any time you can fit it in! Early morning workouts will help you move "back" in time, if you need to wake up earlier than usual. Afternoon or evening exercise will help you stay up later. But any "daytime" exercise gives your internal clock the message, "It's daytime now, and I am active and alert."

Stay healthy.

People often get sick when traveling, thanks to a fatigue-weakened immune system and exposure to new germs. Savvy travelers follow health recommendations for their destinations, wash their hands frequently, and are careful about what they eat. They try to get enough sleep, and avoid stress overload as much as possible.

Reduce travel stress.

Some level of stress seems to be an integral part of travel, and should be anticipated and accommodated rather than ignored. Exert some control over your schedule if possible, and work with your body, rather than against it. Schedule meetings for when you are most likely to feel alert. Reduce your early morning or late evening meetings, if these coincide with 3 a.m. home time. Give yourself enough time for sleep and rest. If you repeatedly travel to the same locations, find hotels that are as quiet and restful as possible. Use earplugs if accommodations are noisy.

If travel stress is a problem, develop some stress reduction strategies. Some travelers learn breathing exercises, meditation techniques, or yoga exercises that help them relax. A relaxing bedtime routine can help you unwind from a busy day and sleep more soundly.

Eat well.

Frequent flyers must learn to make good choices in restaurants, to avoid the overeating that leads to fatigue and weight gain. High protein breakfasts and lunches help you feel more alert, while some carbohydrate in the evening can help you sleep. Consume plenty of fiber, fruits, and vegetables, if available. Judicious use of caffeine can help you wake up at your new morning time, but too much caffeine will make falling asleep at the end of the day more difficult. Limit alcohol, which can increase feelings of jet lag, and lower your resistance to illness.

How Can I Quit Smoking?
Understanding Nicotine Withdrawal

Most of us started smoking when we were young. We knew smoking could cause health problems down the road, but that road seemed awfully long, and those health problems far, far away. More important then was bonding with friends and being cool. Perhaps smoking gave us a distinction and definition we needed back then.

Now we have traveled a ways down the road, and we have seen acquaintances, friends, and perhaps even ourselves, coping with smoking-related illness. We understand more clearly the health consequences of smoking: greater risks of heart disease, cancer, and emphysema. We know about chronic bronchitis, smoker's cough, and recurring colds. Our friends and families are nagging and scolding, joking and cajoling. Enough, we say, let's quit!

Why do some smokers have a harder time quitting than others?

No one knows why some people have little trouble quitting while others struggle for years and make many attempts to quit smoking before they are successful. Many factors are involved. One of the most important is how dependent your body has become on nicotine. In general, the longer you have been a smoker and the more cigarettes you smoke per day, the greater the chance that quitting will be difficult.

Your personal situation may affect how hard it is for you to quit. For example, if your close friends smoke and you are often in places and situations where people are smoking, it may be more challenging for you to kick the habit. If you smoke to take a break from work, you will need to find new ways to take a break and relax. People recovering from an addiction to alcohol or other drugs may find quitting especially difficult. If smoking has helped them through recovery from a more serious addiction, they may be worried about relapse.

Some people may have a hard time quitting because nicotine withdrawal symptoms are especially troublesome for them. These symptoms include not only strong cravings for cigarettes, but emotion symptoms as well, such as depression, anger, irritability, tension, and anxiety. Some people have difficulty concentrating and feel more restless than usual. Difficulty sleeping, increased hunger, and weight gain can also occur during nicotine withdrawal.

What happens during nicotine withdrawal? What causes these symptoms?

The physical and psychological effects of nicotine are not totally understood, but scientists do know that nicotine has powerful effects on our bodies and brains. Nicotine affects many brain chemicals, called neurotransmitters, that affect our moods and our emotions. For example, nicotine may disrupt the regulation of serotonin, the neurotransmitter affected by many antidepressants. Like other strongly addictive drugs (nicotine is as chemically addictive as heroin), nicotine causes changes in brain chemistry that lead to powerful cravings and emotional distress when the drug is withdrawn.

What are some ways to cope with feelings of stress during quitting?

Since negative feelings are the main reason people begin smoking again after they have tried to quit, it is very important for people who want to quit to figure out ways to reduce the stress of quitting. Many people find that smoking cessation programs are extremely helpful. Check with your doctor to find one near you. These programs help you design a quit-smoking strategy that will work for you.

Studies have found that people who exercise regularly have better success quitting smoking than non-exercisers. Exercise can relieve feelings of depression, anxiety, irritability, and tension. Exercise helps combat the negative health effects of smoking, especially by reducing risk for heart disease. Regular physical activity improves sleep quality and helps to prevent or reduce the weight gain that sometimes occurs when people quit smoking.

What kind of exercise is best?

If you have had difficulty quitting smoking in the past, consider exercising almost every day for maximal stress reduction. Find some kind of moderately vigorous exercise that is convenient and enjoyable, if possible. Exercise that occurs in a nonsmoking environment, such as a fitness center, can be especially reinforcing. Getting a friend to walk or do some other form of exercise with you can help you stick to your plans to exercise. Check with your doctor to be sure exercise is safe for you, and get some advice from an exercise instructor or personal trainer if you need some exercise advice.

Quit Smoking: Support for Quitters

Quitting smoking is not easy, but the health benefits are well worth the effort. If you have found kicking the habit difficult in the past, try taking a more comprehensive approach this time. Develop healthful habits that support your new smoke-free lifestyle and that can help you manage the stress of quitting. Following are some suggestions.

Exercise regularly.

Studies show that would-be quitters who exercise are twice as likely to succeed as those who do not. Regular physical activity reduces your risk of gaining weight by burning calories and revving up your metabolism. Exercise also provides temporary relief from cigarette cravings. And a good workout improves your mood, which helps to combat the irritability and depression that can occur during the withdrawal period.

Many people who exercise their way through nicotine withdrawal say that exercise helped keep them on track with their resolutions to quit. Making the time to exercise means making your health a priority. When your lifelong health is a priority, a smoke-free lifestyle is more likely to become a habit.

Get support from family and friends.

Spend as much time as you can with people who support your intentions to quit smoking. Have one or two close friends agree to be there for you during the first few weeks when you need a diversion from cigarette cravings. Get a friend to take walks or play sports with you.

Eat right, and get enough sleep.

Relapse is most likely when you are feeling tired and stressed. Fight fatigue by eating well and getting enough sleep, and avoid snacking unless you are truly hungry. Beware of the tendency that some ex-smokers develop to replace cigarettes with chewing. If chewing helps, try crunchy vegetables or sugarless gum. Drink at least four glasses of water a day to prevent fatigue from dehydration.

If you experience difficulty sleeping, follow guidelines typically recommended for insomnia: Exercise regularly, eliminate caffeine from your diet, manage stress and develop a pleasant bedtime routine.

Join a smoking-cessation program.

Call your local chapter of the American Lung Association or your health-care provider to find programs in your area. These programs offer helpful guidelines, encouragement and social support.

Identify smoking triggers.

Smoking-cessation programs can help you identify your personal smoking triggers so you can prevent relapse. You can also do this on your own. Make a list of times when you smoke (or feel like smoking) throughout the day. Is it during your morning cup of coffee? During breaks at work? When you're stressed? Come up with non-smoking alternatives for these times.

If you have quit smoking before, what made you begin again? Learn from your past experiences. Anticipate situations and feelings that might lead to a relapse, and think of ways to get through these times without resuming a life-threatening habit.

Talk to your doctor.

If quitting has been difficult for you in the past, your health-care provider may recommend medication, such as a nicotine patch or antidepressants, to help you quit smoking.

Stay busy.

When cigarette cravings strike, find a diversion. Go out with non-smoking friends. Take yourself to a smoke-free environment like the fitness center or movie theater. If you must stay home, do chores or develop new hobbies that keep your hands busy.

Reward yourself.

Take the money you have saved from not buying cigarettes and treat yourself to something you enjoy. Get a massage, sign up for an exercise class, or hire a personal trainer to help you improve your exercise program.

123 Treat Your Feet: The Importance of Good Footwear

Take a minute to think about the demands we place on our feet. We often cram them into shoes that are too tight (not to mention high heels) and ask them to walk on concrete sidewalks. Then we go to the fitness center. We ask our feet to walk and run for miles, and make them jump up and down for extended periods of time or zigzag like crazy all over a racquetball court. While the healthy foot is a strong, sturdy structure, the repetitive-movement demands of activities such as aerobics, tennis, and basketball can cause problems. That's why we must take the time (and spend the money) to shop for good shoes.

Is special footwear important for exercise?

For many sports and activities, well-fitting shoes that will accommodate the extra demands placed on your feet are essential. Indeed, a good shoe is the most important part of your outfit, so spend your money here and wear your old T-shirts for another year.

The stresses placed on your feet vary from sport to sport. Sport shoe manufacturers analyze the biomechanical demands of a given sport and design shoes to protect your foot from the injuries associated with those movements.

For example, when you run, your feet receive a force that is two to three times your body weight with each step. Running shoes are designed to give your feet extra cushioning for absorbing this shock, especially in the heel. A stiff heel counter and flared heel sole give good support and stability, and, with the arch support, help to prevent the foot from rolling in or out. Padded heels help to protect the Achilles tendon.

Walking shoes also provide support and shock absorption, but are built to accommodate the rolling motion of your foot, rather than a pounding impact. Heel cushioning, arch supports and flexible soles are important. Walking shoes should also help prevent the foot from rolling in or out.

Some activities, such as aerobics, require a repeated up-and-down motion. Aerobics shoes should have good overall support and adequate cushioning. Many activities also require frequent changes in direction. Shoes for these activities should have good overall support to resist twisting of the foot and ankle. Running shoes can be dangerous for activities requiring lateral movement, as you may trip over the flared heel.

When should I get a new pair of sports shoes?

Since good shoes are often expensive, we tend to hang on to them longer than we should. The first thing to go in a sports shoe is usually its shock-absorbing ability, so the shoe may still look fine, but not be performing one of its most important functions. Experts suggest that aerobics and court shoes usually need to be replaced after about 50 to 75 hours of use, and running shoes after about 400 to 500 miles. Heavier people tend to wear out their shoes faster than lighter folks.

To see for yourself if your shoes need replacing, check three things. First, how are you feeling? If you are developing shin splints or other leg and foot pains, try new shoes. Second, try twisting your shoe. Worn out shoes will twist more easily than new ones. And last, try on a new pair of the brand you like, and compare how they feel to your old ones. Better cushion and support? It may be time to buy the new shoes.

I recently bought shoes recommended by my teacher, but they are really not as comfortable as my last pair.

The most common cause of foot problems are ill-fitting shoes, which interfere with the foot's natural structure and function. Many people spend a great deal of time researching which brand of shoes to buy, but do not spend adequate time evaluating whether the shoe is suited to their foot. A high-quality shoe is only worth buying if it fits! Better to buy a lesser-quality shoe that fits well than a poorly fitting high-quality shoe.

Shop for shoes in the late afternoon when your feet are at their largest. One foot is often bigger than the other; measure your feet if you're not sure about yours. Always buy for the bigger foot. The shoes you try on should feel comfortable immediately. Don't plan on shoes stretching with wear. The heel should fit snugly, and the instep should not gape open. The toe box should be wide enough to wiggle all your toes, and the shoe should be as wide as your forefoot.

This last point is often overlooked. Many people think it is normal to push their feet into too-narrow shoes, perhaps believing this is part of the "support" shoes should offer. But unless you have problem feet, your arches give you good support. If you do have problems with a foot structure that does not allow normal movement, a podiatrist can sometimes correct the problem with shoe inserts to change the way your foot works.

Barbara A. Brehm, Ed.D. is a professor of exercise and sport studies at Smith College in Northampton, Massachusetts, where she teaches courses in stress management, nutrition, and health. She has worked as a fitness instructor, personal trainer, lifestyle coach, and fitness program director, and has helped hundreds of people in her classes and other programs become more active.

Dr. Brehm has written about health and fitness for over 25 years. Her specialty is translating exercise and health science for real people, and she writes extensively for fitness professionals. She has received the San Diego County Medical Society Media Award and was a Maggie Award finalist for her regular columns for *Fitness Management*, where she served as a contributing editor. She is the co-author of *Applied Sports Medicine for Coaches* (Lippincott, Williams, and Wilkins) and author of several other books, including *Successful Fitness Motivation Strategies* (Human Kinetics).

About the Author